MODERN
LESSON PLANS IN

Environmental Science

Helen Hoch Kotsonis
and Bill Baker

PARKER PUBLISHING COMPANY, INC. / WEST NYACK, N.Y.

Library of Congress Cataloging in Publication Data

Kotsonis, Helen Hoch, (date)
    Modern lesson plans in environmental science.

    Includes bibliographies.
    1. Ecology--Study and teaching (Secondary)
2. Environmental health--Study and teaching.
3. Pollution--Study and teaching (Secondary)
I. Baker, Bill, joint author. II. Title.
QH541.2.K68   301.31'07'12   72-3956
ISBN 0-13-594978-5

Printed in the United States of America

We dedicate this book to
Helen and Michael Baker and Sophie and John Hoch,
our dear, delightful, and wonderful parents,
as a fitting tribute for everything they have done for us.

How Lesson Plans in Environmental Science Will Help the Teacher

America is being seriously affected by pollutants from coast to coast. The Great Lakes are poisoned by nitrates and industrial wastes, while strip mining in Appalachia causes acid to drip into the rivers and streams. Noise pollution is contributing to an increase in hearing loss and heart damage. Each year man adds more than 800 million tons of pollutants to the atmosphere. The exhaust from automobiles and other vehicles causes over sixty percent of the air pollution in our cities. The increase of carbon dioxide in our atmosphere from these exhausts will change the temperature of the earth, and could eventually lead to floods or the formation of another ice age. The number of babies born every twenty-five minutes in the United States is enough to populate an entire city. The accumulation of pesticides in the human body can lead to a variety of serious ailments and diseases.

From these few examples, it is evident that the study of ecology and the entire concept of environmental science must be included in the contemporary secondary school curriculum. The purpose of this book is to help you to teach the basic tenets of ecology. To be totally informed about our environment and the many ecological crises confronting it would be impossible for one person, so complex and far-reaching are the effects of man's technology on the earth. This book, therefore, will serve the teacher as a comprehensive sourcebook of some of the environmentalist's concerns, how best to present them to their students,

7

together with valuable suggestions for solving some of the problems besetting the environment. This book will further help you
develop in your students the ability to ask the right questions
about what is going on in their environment, and to help them do
their part to protect it.

Environmental science information currently available to the
teacher comes from such varied sources as newspaper and magazine articles, television and radio news programs, teach-ins and
seminars, pamphlets from the many diverse national, state, and
local organizations, and other similarly assorted sources. As a
result of this great diversity of source materials, a great deal of the
teacher's valuable time would be required to research and develop
lessons in environmental science. Thus, this book is unique
because it brings the teacher *complete* plans that can be used right
from the book for teaching the various concepts of environmental
science.

This book can be used by all who teach biology, general
science, and hygiene. Our aim has been to develop a series of
lesson plans which brings together the most recent information
and innovative techniques. Every aspect of each lesson has been
successfully tested in actual classroom and laboratory use. These
lessons offer the science teacher concrete activities, lessons, materials, and information specifically designed to stimulate student
interest in their natural environment. This material will supply the
teacher with a guide that is both practical and applicable to the
classroom situation; and provides valuable ideas about dealing with
the basic concepts of environmental science.

We have included in each lesson:

1. Appropriate demonstrations and experiments dealing
   with the unit to be studied
2. Laboratory procedures for students
3. Suggested laboratory preparations, including equipment
   and time requirements for the teacher
4. Alternate methods of presentation to help clarify any
   difficult concept the lesson may include
5. Appropriate illustrations, charts, and diagrams to further clarify the lesson
6. Pertinent facts to be emphasized
7. Suggested questions for a possible quiz

8. Lists of audio-visual materials and projects appropriate for each particular lesson
9. Suggested bibliography for *both* teacher and students

Both beginning and experienced teachers alike will find these lessons helpful in organizing an effective curriculum on a current and pressing topic.

Contents

Lesson 1 — Water Pollution — 17

Develops a working definition of water pollution, including its causes and effects, using a laboratory approach to the problems involved and derives possible methods of solution.

Lesson 2 — Air Pollution — 25

Uses knowledge of the respiratory system and various types of air contaminants to determine the harmful effects of air pollutuants on nonliving materials, and, through experiments on fruit flies, the harmful effects to living tissue.

Lesson 3 — Thermal Pollution — 33

Determines the temperature range of simple plants and the effect of thermal pollution on enzyme activities through laboratory experiment, and postulates the effects of such pollution on the survival of living organisms.

Lesson 4 — Noise Pollution — 39

Uses knowledge of auditory functioning to explain the harmful effects of loud noises on the human ear as determined from an experiment in which various types of sounds found in the home and school are compared.

Lesson 5 — Pesticide Pollution — 45

Conceptualizes alternatives to the use of pesticides for the control of insects and other pests from an understanding of their life cycles and characteristics.

Lesson 6 — Pollution and Food Additives — 53

Explores the uses of food additives, the reasons for their use, and the harmful effects they can produce in human tissue; and deter-

The Dynamics
of Pollution

UNIT 1

LESSON 1

Water Pollution

Lesson time: 45 minutes
Laboratory time: 45-90 minutes

Aim

To develop a working definition of water pollution, including its causes and effects, using a laboratory approach to the problems involved and deriving possible methods of solution.

Materials

mixed culture of Protists
$AgNo_3$, and $Ba(C_2H_3O_2)_2$
dilute NaOH, HCl, HNO_3
concentrated NH_4OH, H_2SO_4

Planned Lesson

1. *What Is Water Pollution?* The teacher might begin the study of water pollution with an introductory assignment in which students are asked to collect and bring in current news articles on water pollution. These may be made into a bulletin board type display and used at an appropriate time, as the study progresses.

The information obtained from these sources can be used to develop a working definition of water pollution. References can then be used to determine the microbiological definition of water pollution. *Why is oxygen depletion the only characteristic considered in the microbiologist's definition? How does it differ from the layman's definition? Is water pollution a recent development?* The teacher can here point out that water pollution is older than recorded history.

2. *Urbanization and Water Pollution.* The class should consider the various naturally occurring cycles which tend to eliminate impurities. Specifically, they will need to be concerned with the biochemical activities of bacteria as well as with dilution, sedimentation, and sunlight. *Can you give a brief explantion of the effects of increase or decrease of dilution, sedimentation, or sunlight on purification? As self-purification requires a varying amount of distance of flow and time, what is the relationship to population increase and urbanization?* Students should be encouraged throughout their study of the environment to look at the total picture. They will need to go beyond a consideration of a single community. *What is happening in the whole region? Why is this important?*

3. *Possible Solutions.* The discussion may logically turn to solutions for the problem. This provides a good point at which to consider the widely held theory that current technology exists to correct such difficulties. Students might be asked to do reports on this topic. They should be encouraged to seek out data so that they can determine the extent to which water pollution technology has been developed. It should be emphasized that scientists do not have all the answers. Students might set up a panel discussion using the information they find on the current limits and feasibility of today's technology, to consider a question such as, *"What is a tolerable level of water pollution?"*

4. *Student Activities.* For the interested student or the advanced class, the teacher might suggest readings dealing with the more technical aspects of measuring pollution in terms of oxygen criteria. B.O.D., biochemical oxygen demand, D.O., dissolved oxygen, and coliform density might all be subjects for reports or possible field trips to laboratories which monitor these. For activities concerning water-borne diseases, the teacher might use Lesson 25, Infectious Diseases.

5. *Laboratory Activities.* The observation of microbial life

in a drop of water could serve as a focal point for a laboratory activity. Water samples should be collected from various sources. Students should be reminded to use good technique as to proper labeling of collecting jars. Labels should include place, time and date of collection, as well as distance from shoreline and depth at which the sample was taken, if appropriate. Before collection begins, a discussion should be held concerning possible sources (such as tap water, water from a nearby hydrant, puddles, ponds, lakes, streams, rivers) and possible sampling containers. In the laboratory, wet mounts should be prepared and microorganisms observed with the microscope. Each organism should be carefully drawn, labeled, and identified. The teacher can provide references for student use from the bibliography at the end of this lesson.

A. Preparing simple wet mounts. A number of cells and tissues can be mounted in a drop of fluid, usually water. Water is an excellent mounting fluid for living materials. Some difficulties to be considered include the rapid evaporation of water, rapid loss of oxygen from the water and the entrapment of air under the tissue. Mineral oil may also be used. The visibility of some cell parts is better in mineral oil than in water, and tissues remain alive for longer periods of time. Some materials which can be prepared as wet mounts include protozoa, onion epidermis, elodea leaves, cheek cells, and nonliving materials.

The procedure is quite simple. A drop of water is placed on a clean glass slide, and the material to be mounted is placed in it. A very small amount of material should be used so that light can pass through. A cover slip should than be placed over the specimen. (It is important that no air be trapped under the cover slip.) The cover slip should be placed on the slide so that one edge is touching the slide, with the remainder of the cover slip held away from the slide, as illustrated in Figure 1-1. The cover slip should then be slowly lowered so that no air is trapped beneath it.

In order to insure that microorganisms are observed, a mixed culture should be available in the laboratory. This may be prepared by the teacher or student, or may be obtained from a supply house, such as General Biological Supply House, Inc., 8200 South Hoyne Avenue, Chicago, Illinois 60620; or Carolina Biological Supply Co., Burlington, North Carolina 27215.

B. Preparing a mixed culture. If you prefer, you can have

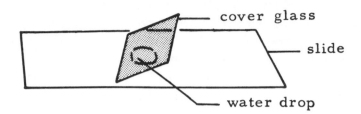

cover glass

slide

water drop

Figure 1-1. Cover Slip Technique

your students collect these organisms themselves. On their own time, such as on weekends or after school, have students locate a nearby pond, lake, stream, or even a ditch which contains water. Have them take along an empty container or jar with a stopper, and ask them to collect a sample of water, surface scum, or bottom ooze, all of which may contain cysts or motile stages of various protozoa. After these samples have been brought to the laboratory, the students can develop cultures by adding grass, leaves, or bits of boiled lettuce to a jar or other suitable container, and adding enough water to more than cover the material. This should then be allowed to stand in a warm place away from direct sunlight.

A follow-up activity can be used to study the chemical content of these water samples. Student volunteers can prepare the reagent solutions: dilute NaOH, HCl, HNO_3, $AgNO_3$, $Ba(C_2H_3O_2)_2$, concentrated NH_4OH, and H_2SO_4. Exact molarities are not significant unless a quantitative analysis is to be done. Figures 1-2 and 1-3 can be duplicated and used as a laboratory guide.

For interested students the teacher can recommend *Standard Methods for the Examination of Water and Waste Water*. This can be used as a source for more detailed analysis for advanced laboratory groups.

6. *Field Activities.* Field trips can be arranged in consultation with local, state, and federal agencies, citizens' groups, or nearby colleges and universities. Points of interest could include

Cation	6 M NaOH	Excess 14.8 M NH_4OH	0.3 M HCL
Pb^{+2}	$Pb(OH)_2$ (s), white	$Pb(OH)_2$ (s), white	$PbCl_2$ (s), white
Hg_2^{+2}	HgO (s), yellow and Hg (s), black	$Hg(NH_2)Cl$ (s), (If Cl⁻ ions present)	Hg_2Cl_2 (s), white
Cu^{+2}	$Cu(OH)_2$ (s), blue	$(Cu(NH_3)_4)^{+2}$(s), azure blue	No reaction
Fe^{+3}	$Fe(OH)_3$ (s), rust-brown	$Fe(OH)_3$ (s), rust-brown	No reaction
Ca^{+2}	$Ca(OH)_2$ (s), white	No reaction	No reaction

Figure 1-2. Products Formed in the Reaction of Aqueous Solutions of Cations with Various Reagents.

neighboring ponds, lakes, streams, riverbanks, sewage plants, reservoirs, state parks, fish and game preserves, and the various laboratories involved in water analysis. Most of these sources also provide guest speakers, films, or other materials suitable for in-school or community programs.

What Can You Do?

1. Have your parents support local and state water pollution control agencies. This can usually be accomplished by voting for clean water bonds.
2. Tell your parents to actively support measures which are designed to achieve water quality.
3. Have your parents and relatives write to local, state, or federal representatives to enact legislation that will cut down on the amount of pollution poured into our waters by various industrial sources.
4. Go on a field trip to your local water treatment plant. While there, you will not only learn how it operates, but

Anion	Litmus	Dilute HNO_3	$AgNO_3$	$Ba(C_2H_3O_2)_2$	MnO_4^- - H^+	Concentrated H_2SO_4
Cl^-	No reaction	No reaction	White precipitate, insoluble in H^+	No reaction	Forms Cl_2; Mn^{+2} colorless solution	Pungent gas; fumes in moist air (HCl)
SO_4^{-2}	No reaction	No reaction	White precipitate, soluble in H^+	White precipitate, insoluble in H^+	No reaction	No reaction
PO_4^{-3}	Turns blue	No reaction	Yellow precipitate, soluble in H^+	White precipitate, soluble in H^+	No reaction	No reaction
CO_3^{-2}	Turns blue	Forms CO_2 (g)+ H_2O	White precipitate, soluble in H^+	White precipitate, soluble in H	No reaction; CO_2 (g) from H^+ present	Effervesces; CO_2 (g) from H^+ present

Figure 1-3. Reactions of Anions with Various Reagents.

also what you and your family can do to make the operation of this plant more effective.

Pertinent Facts

1. Microbiologically, water pollution is a depletion of oxygen.
2. In lay terms, pollution encompasses the presence of any contaminant in water sources.
3. Self-purification involves the action of bacteria, dilution, sedimentation, and sunlight.
4. With an increase in urbanization, the self-purification of water cannot occur effectively because of lack of time and increased concentration of effluent.
5. Effluent is the material which leaves a sewage plant after treatment and processing; its purity depending upon the effectiveness of treatment.
6. Anions are negatively charged particles; cations are positively charged particles.

Possible Quiz

1. Compare the microbiologist's definition of water pollution with the one developed in class.
2. Explain how bacterial action affects water purification. What role do dilution, sedimentation, and sunlight have in the purification process?
3. Why is it essential to consider the regional pollution picture when planning a local pollution control project?
4. Is there a prevailing type of organism in most samples of water observed? How can you account for this?
5. What ions did you find in your water sample? Give a possible explanation for their presence.

READINGS

Baker, Bill, and Helen Kotsonis, *Modern Lesson Plans for the Biology Teacher.* West Nyack, New York: Parker Publishing Co., Inc., 1970.

Berg, Gerald, *Transmission of Viruses by the Water Route.* New York: Interscience Publishers, 1967.

Bruce, F.E., "Water Supply, Sanitation, and Disposal of Waste Matter" in W. Hobson, ed., *Theory and Practice of Public Health.* London: Oxford University Press, 1961.

Ehlers, V.M., and E.W. Steel, *Municipal and Rural Sanitation,* 6th edition. New York: McGraw-Hill, Inc., 1965.

Hutton, Wilbert, *General Chemistry Laboratory Text with Qualitative Analysis.* Columbus, Ohio: Charles E. Merrill Co., 1968.

Standard Methods for the Examination of Water and Waste Water, 12th Edition. Albany, New York: Boyd Printing Co., Inc., 1965.

FILMS

"A Day at the Dump." 15 minutes, sound, color, free. Environmental Control Commission, 12720 Twinbrook Parkway, Rockville, Maryland 20852.

"Water Pollution." 15 minutes, color, sound, $8.00. Encyclopedia Brittanica Educational Corporation, 425 North Michigan Avenue, Chicago, Ill. 60611.

LESSON 2

Air Pollution

Lesson time: 45 minutes
Laboratory time: 45-90 minutes

Aim

To use knowledge of the respiratory system and various types of air contaminants to determine the harmful effects of air pollutants on nonliving materials, and, through experiments on fruit flies, the harmful effects to living tissue.

Materials

lima bean seedlings	soil
hand lens	graph paper
test tubes	glass funnels
large-mouthed jars	rubber tubing
fine cheesecloth	sulfur
gasoline	agar
Drosophila virilis	

Planned Lesson

1. *Mechanics of Respiration.* A study of air pollution can begin with a review of human and animal respiration, or, if preferred, this study might immediately follow such a unit. It would be valuable for the students to have a grasp of the mechanics of respiration, both at the lungs and at the cells. They

25

should also be able to briefly describe the process of breathing. *How does air get into our lungs? Why is the mucus coating of the lungs important?*

2. *What Is Air Pollution?*   Students can be asked to list various contaminants found in air. *What are the most common pollutants in your area? Are the pollutants the same in every area?* Student lists can be expanded to include sources of contaminants, possible effects on plant and animal tissues, and effects on surfaces exposed to contaminated air. Class discussion can logically lead to a working definition of air pollution. This definition should include the idea that air pollution is the presence of substances in the air in quantities large enough to interfere with comfort, safety, and health.

3. *How Does It Develop?*   *What are some common sources of pollutants?* Using the student developed lists, the exhausts from cars, planes, and other vehicles, the burning of fuel, industrial processes, the burning of waste, construction projects, movement of polluted air masses, natural phenomena, as well as other sources, can be discussed. *How can the sources of these pollutants be controlled or eliminated? What controls have been established in your community? How effective are they?*

4. *Some Common Pollutants.*   The student lists can again be used to consider some specific pollutants. *What are some pollutants usually found in gaseous form?* Among those likely to be listed are sulfur dioxide, carbon monoxide, hydrocarbons, ammonia, oxides of nitrogen, organic acids, and tetraethyl lead. *Which ones are likely to be particulate in nature?* Soot, ash, dust, pollen, and various chemicals in powdered form should be mentioned. *What effect does pollution have on buildings, clothing, and other nonliving materials?* It might be mentioned that researchers are attempting to formulate compounds which could be used to protect the façades of historical monuments. As part of the investigation into air pollution, students can determine the various methods that are in use for detecting and measuring the concentrations of pollutants in the air. They should have little difficulty locating periodicals with up-to-date information, or they can be encouraged to contact local, state, or federal offices which conduct such tests to tabulate this information. This may also lead to an invitation for a source person to come to visit the group or even for a group field trip.

5. *Physiology of Air Pollution.* The effects of these contaminants on the body can now be discussed. A review of the uses
of oxygen in the cell would be very helpful. Here the teacher
might mention that the pigment, hemoglobin, in red blood cells
carries the oxygen to the cells (oxyhemoglobin), and carbon
dioxide away from them (carboxyhemoglobin). A capsule discussion of the role of hemoglobin in oxygen transport will be very
helpful in studying the physiology of carbon monoxide poisoning.
The concept that hemoglobin has a higher affinity for carbon
monoxide than for oxygen should be stressed. *Why is high
pressure oxygen in hyperbaric chambers used to treat carbon
monoxide poisoning?* The student lists can be once again used
here. Student committees can be organized to collect information
on health problems caused by contaminants in the air. This is an
excellent means for developing problem-solving techniques and
initiative. The teacher should serve only as a guide and source of
encouragement. Suggested sources would probably include: local
physicians, hospitals, medical schools, the various national founda-
tions such as the Heart Association or Cancer Society, local, state,
and federal public health facilities and research-oriented laboratories such as the Memorial Sloan-Kettering Cancer Center of New
York City. *What is the physiology of black lung disease? Why does
air pollution complicate the problem of respiratory disease? Why
is smoking a health hazard?*
    6. *Student Projects.* A natural consequence of student
activities is the development of a bulletin board type display for
the edification of the entire school. Ideally this should be set up in
a centrally located area of the school. This display could include a
large chart which incorporates the information from the individual
student lists, an attractively arranged collection of pamphlets,
names and addresses of organizations involved in fighting pollution, and perhaps some helpful hints related to what the individual
can do to help. The interest generated by such a project might
very well lead to a full scale program. This could be a day long
activity involving speakers, films, and demonstrations which could
further lead to an ongoing class or school-wide activity. Any such
activity will require careful planning by students and discreet
guidance by faculty.
    7. *Laboratory Activities.* Several feasible activities related
to air pollution can be effectively developed in the laboratory.

Students can use a stop watch to determine how long they can hold their breath. This can serve as an excellent illustration of how important air is to life.

In order to determine the amount of particulate "fallout" in various neighborhoods of the community, the following will be effective. In class, the group can prepare sheets of graph paper (preferably with a tinted rather than a white background) by spraying the surface lightly with hair spray or aerosol glue. The sheets can then be taped to the window sill. Conditions may be varied for each. Encourage the students to develop alternates such as the window open from the bottom an inch, a foot; closed; open only at the top; paper on outside sill, and so forth. After some agreed upon time interval, all sheets should be removed and observed. Using a hand lens will simplify the counting of particles in a square. They should count five squares, perhaps the center and corner squares, and average. The tinted paper will make observation easier if the particles include soap or other light-colored material. To compare varying environmental conditions, students can take graph paper home and repeat the procedure being careful to record all pertinent data. *Is there a difference in concentration of particulate matter from one area to another? Can you account for this?*

A study of the genetic effects of air pollution can also serve as an excellent means for developing laboratory techniques in an interesting and informative manner.

Since live materials are being used, it would be wise to order Drosophila at least one month in advance. Divide the class into four groups. Each group will need four test tubes with ten pairs of flies each as a control; four test tubes with ten pairs of flies each to be treated five to ten minutes daily with the fumes of burning gasoline; four test tubes with ten pairs of flies each to be treated five to ten minutes daily with the fumes from burning sulfur.

Each test tube should contain about an inch of nutrient medium. Most supply houses include a booklet giving instruction in all aspects of care and handling of fruit flies, or students may use various source books, including Baker and Kotsonis, *Modern Lesson Plans for the Biology Teacher.* The test tubes should be covered with cheesecloth fastened with rubber bands or string.

Two empty metal cans (10-15 ounce size) can be used as stoves by punching holes in the bottom. The cans should be inverted over a suitable container such as a pyrex beaker, so that gasoline or sulfur can be burned to produce the "air pollution" for the experiment. A glass funnel placed on top of each can will serve to collect the fumes produced. Rubber tubing attached to the narrow end of the funnel will channel the fumes to a large-mouth jar containing the four test tubes of experimental flies. The jar must be large enough so that the cap can be tightly closed. The cap should have two holes punched in it to allow passage of two pieces of rubber tubing. The rubber tubing from the funnel should pass through one of these holes, while a second piece of rubber tubing should pass through the second hole with its end attached to a faucet aspirator. Any gaps between tubes and openings in the cap should be sealed with petroleum jelly, liquid paraffin, or some other suitable material. The faucet aspirator will serve to draw the fumes into the jar.

One week will probably be sufficient to induce genetic changes. In preparation for the observation of the flies and the offspring, each group of flies should be transferred to test tubes containing fresh media. All groups should remain undisturbed for three to five days at which time each group of adult flies should be transferred again to test tubes with fresh media. The pupae should be observed using a hand lens or dissecting microscope. A clear plastic ruler, small scale graph paper, or similar device will help to compare body lengths of pupae. All such observations should be tabulated. Students should also record approximate hatching time. *How do controls and experimental flies compare? What is significant about your observations?*

What Can You Do?

1. Have your parents and family fight for legislation designed to limit the maximum allowable level of air pollutants leaving any industrial or power plant in your neighborhood.

2. Make certain the family car gets a tune-up periodically. This will not only make it run more efficiently, but will

also cut down on the number and amount of byproducts entering the atmosphere.
3. Stop smoking.
4. Use an electric lawnmower or a hand operated one. Do not use gas-driven mowers or other garden equipment.
5. Set up a compost pile in your backyard for leaves and grass cuttings. Burning of leaves adds to the pollution of our air.

Pertinent Facts

1. Breathing is the mechanical process of bringing in and releasing air from the body while respiration is the transfer of gases at the lungs and cells.
2. Large transport planes such as those of the SST category make a significant contribution to air pollution as do most aspects of modern life.
3. Not only are living tissues harmed by air pollution, but buildings, clothing, and other nonliving materials are also damaged.
4. Exposure to sulfur dioxide fumes causes premature aging in Drosophila virilis.
5. Exposure to oxidized hydrocarbons (burning gasoline fumes) causes decreased longevity in Drosophila virilis.

Possible Quiz

1. Briefly describe the differences between breathing and respiration.
2. List some common air pollutants, possible sources of them, and the effects they have on living tissue.
3. What is significant about the fact that hemoglobin has a greater affinity for carbon monoxide than for oxygen or carbon dioxide?
4. Is the pollution of air a necessary consequence of our style of life?
5. What are the specific effects of sulfur dioxide and oxidized hydrocarbons on living tissue?

READINGS

Anderson, D.O., and B.G. Ferris, Jr., "Community Studies of the Health Effects of Air Pollution: A Critique," *Air Pollution Control Association Journal* 15:587, 1965.

Baker, Bill, and Helen Kotsonis, *Modern Lesson Plans for the Biology Teacher.* West Nyack, New York, Parker Publishing Co., Inc., 1970.

Goldsmith, J.R., "Air Pollution Epidemiology," *Archives of Environmental Health* 18:516, 1969.

McDermott, Walsh, "Air Pollution and Public Health," *Scientific American,* October, 1961, p. 206.

Meethan, A.R., *Atmosphere Pollution,* 3rd ed. New York: Macmillan,1964.

"The Polluted Air," *Time Magazine,* Vol. 89, No. 4, January 27, 1967.

Winklestein, W., "Air Pollution Respiratory Function Study," 8th AMA Conference on Air Pollution. Los Angeles, March, 1966.

FILMS

"Air Pollution: Take a Deep Deadly Breath." 54 minutes, sound, color, $35.00. McGraw-Hill, ABC Documentary, Film Rental Offices, 330 West 42nd Street, New York, N.Y. 10018.

"Air Pollution." 15 minutes, sound, color, $8.00. Encyclopedia Brittanica, Educational Corporation, 425 North Michigan Ave., Chicago, Illinois 60611.

"Ill Winds on a Sunny Day." 29 minutes, sound, color, free. National Medical Audio-Visual Center, Station K, Atlanta, Georgia 30324.

LESSON 3

Thermal Pollution

Lesson time: 45 minutes
Laboratory time: 90 minutes

Aim

To determine the temperature range of simple plants and the effect of thermal pollution on enzyme activities through laboratory experiment, and to postulate the effects of such pollution on the survival of living organisms.

Materials

liver	test tubes and rack
hydrogen peroxide	stirring rod
distilled water	sodium hydroxide
aquarium	adjustable fish tank heater
aquarium plants	metal ice cube trays

Planned Lesson

1. *What Is Thermal Pollution?*   Having previously considered water and air pollution, students should be aware of some of the problems of changes in heat levels. In this lesson, the problem can be directly attacked.

The term "thermal pollution" conjures up in students' minds the local consequence of heat from the generation of electrical power. While the warming of rivers, lakes, and bays by this means is a matter of concern, it is but one aspect of a more fundamental problem. It should be pointed out that *all* human activities, from metabolism to plowing a field, to driving a car, result in the dissipation of heat.

2. *What Are Some Sources of Heat Which Affect Water Temperature?* Students will most likely mention atomic power plants because they are so often in the news. Manufacturing plants will also be listed, but they frequently overlook the sun as a source of heat.

Students should understand that water can absorb a great amount of heat before its temperature begins to rise (specific heat). They can relate this to "a watched pot never boils." *What is the basis for this expression?* They can also consider it in terms of human physiology. As, for example, the ability of water to absorb a great amount of energy in cells, and yet maintain a constant body temperature; or, its role as perspiration.

The production of energy in the Kreb's cycle can be discussed in terms of water's characteristic of good heat conductivity and slow temperature change. Students can then relate these to the functioning of the cell and of the entire organism. *Why are we called warm-blooded? Why aren't some areas of the body much warmer than others, even though there is greater cellular activity (and therefore more heat) in some areas than in others?* It will be necessary to stress that even though some organisms do not have a specific body temperature and are therefore called cold-blooded, they can function only within a specific temperature range.

It would be worthwhile to explore the nature and functioning of enzymes at this point. Students might be asked to read about the protein nature of enzymes and the limits on their functioning. Critical to this study will be the narrow range of pH and temperature within which these crucial chemicals operate. A simple laboratory activity can be used to develop an understanding of enzyme functioning. This could also be used to relate with chemical water pollution as it alters pH.

The Effect of Temperature. Place some liver (crushed) in the bottom of a test tube and stand it in a boiling water bath for about 5 minutes. Then add about 1 ml of fresh hydrogen peroxide to the boiled liver. Observe and record your results.

Take two test tubes an'd add 1 ml of hydrogen peroxide to

each. Place one of the test tubes in a warm water bath (37°C) and the other in an ice water bath for about five minutes. Then remove both tubes from their water baths and place a small piece of liver in each. Compare the rates of the reactions.

The Effect of pH. Into each of three clean test tubes place a small piece of liver. Use a stirring rod and some sand to crush the liver. Add 2 ml of distilled water to the first; 2 ml of sodium hydroxide to the second; and 2 ml of hydrogen peroxide into each tube. Observe and record results.

This laboratory exercise should help focus the student's analysis of thermal pollution on enzyme activities. As they have already reviewed the role of enzymes in cellular functioning, they can now draw conclusions concerning the results of changes in environmental temperature. *When organisms, such as fish, die from thermal pollution, what is one likely reason?*

Student reports can consider the dilution of water as a means of reducing thermal pollution. *Is this a likely possibility? Has the temperature of the oceans changed?*

As in every area of ecological study, speakers and field trips can be used to develop the topic further. A great many citizens' groups have been organized to deal with nuclear power plants, and other sources of thermal pollution. Power companies provide speakers and films. The teacher may wish to plan a field trip to a nearby nuclear power plant or to a manufacturing plant. In many industries, films are available which illustrate the many different manufacturing processes. The teacher can contact local factories to check on the availability of such films. The showing of the film can serve as an introduction to a visit to a plant.

3. *Power Needs vs. Pollution Problems.* *Do nuclear plants pollute? If so, to what extent?* The students should be encouraged to consider the idea that "all power pollutes," since it will be considered again and again from different aspects. They should also be encouraged to follow through on the topic by reading various articles on the subject, and from their own personal experiences. Perhaps they might establish a school Ecology Bulletin or Ecology Bulletin Board for which they would be responsible.

4. *Laboratory Activity.* To test the temperature range of

simple plants, a laboratory project can be developed using small containers, such as aquaria and adjustable fish tank heaters. Students should be encouraged to develop their own procedure. Simple aquarium plants such as Elodea, Sagittaria, or Valissneria may be used. One should serve as a control at room temperature, while other plants of the same species can be placed in tanks of varying temperatures. All tanks should have the same amount of light. *What is the range of temperature within which the experimental organism survives?* Most living organisms can survive only within rather narrow ranges of temperature. *Why is this? If one or several of the plants or animals in an aquatic environment is killed by thermal pollution, what possible effects will this have on the entire aquatic community?*

Mention should be made that increases in temperature will decrease the amount of gas which can be dissolved in a liquid. This can be illustrated by a simple laboratory activity in which two metal containers (such as ice cube trays) are filled with water, one at room temperature, and one with boiling water. The trays should be placed in a refrigerator and the time recorded. The trays should then be checked at half hour intervals until evidence of freezing is seen. The time interval can then be reduced to fifteen minutes, until one tray has solidified. *Which tray solidified first? Why? Why does a bottle of warm soda bubble over more easily than a cold one when opened?* The phenomenon can now be related to the need for dissolved oxygen by aquatic organisms.

It can also be mentioned that increased temperatures cause chemical reactions to occur at a faster rate. This then means that more oxygen is needed to keep up with the rate. *What, then, is the total effect of increased thermal pollution of water?*

Student reports might investigate some ways in which thermal pollution can be controlled. *Does thermal pollution exist in your area? What methods are used to control it?*

What Can You Do?

1. Press for and support legislation designed to force power and electrical plants to cool water from these plants before letting it run into rivers, lakes, and streams.

2. Have your parents form or join a citizens committee to insure that local power plants do not add "hot" water to natural water sources.

Pertinent Facts

1. All human activities result in the dissipation of heat.
2. Most people think of thermal pollution as the production of waste heat from the generation of electrical power.
3. Increased temperatures cause chemical reactions to occur at faster rates.
4. Since enzymes function best within narrow temperature ranges, any change in temperature will alter enzyme action.
5. Most organisms function within a narrow temperature range because the enzymes they contain function within a narrow temperature range.

Possible Quiz

1. Define the term "thermal pollution." How many causes of thermal pollution can you identify in your area?
2. Explain why most organisms function only within narrow temperature ranges.
3. How would thermal pollution affect the basic metabolism of aquatic organisms?
4. Describe the effect of temperature, pH, and particle size on the rate of enzyme action.
5. Explain the relationship between increased temperature and the amount of oxygen present in a lake or stream.

READINGS

Carter, L.J. "Warm Water Irrigation: An Answer to Thermal Pollution." *Science,* 165:478-80, 1969.

Clark, John R., "Thermal Pollution and Aquatic Life." *Scientific American,* 220:18, 1969.

Cole, La Mont C., "Thermal Pollution." *Bioscience,* 19:989-92, 1969.

FILMS

Films on thermal pollution may be obtained by contacting the public relations office of a local manufacturing company, power plant, or industry. They will also arrange for guest speakers to come to your class to discuss the various aspects of this problem.

LESSON 4

Noise Pollution

Lesson time: 45-90 minutes
Laboratory time: 45 minutes

Aim

To use knowledge of auditory functioning to explain the harmful effects of loud noises on the human ear as determined from an experiment in which various types of sounds found in the home and school are compared.

Materials

> tuning fork
> film
> cotton
> sound survey meters

Planned Lesson

1. *Why Do We Take Noise for Granted?* A classroom activity can be the development of a list of noise sources in the vicinity of the school. Students will be somewhat surprised at the list. *Would we be comfortable in an atmosphere of silence?* The teacher might here introduce some of the studies involving soundproof rooms and human volunteers. Students will be interested to learn that we react with a number of problems and

psychological changes if we are kept in silence for prolonged periods. They might want to discuss some of the theories which suggest that the brain needs the stimulation of various sounds. Interested students can research this further, and give an oral report to the class.

2. *What Is Noise Pollution?* This can develop into an interesting discussion which again can lead students to read about professional opinions and definitions.

A home project assignment might involve having students observe their households for a few days and to list sources of noise. The class as a whole can then decide which of these noises constitutes noise pollution.

A field trip to an airport can be arranged so that students can see the methods used to reduce jet noise and to protect workers from ear damage. *How much noise is required before damage to the ears or other body tissues occurs?* (Physics textbooks can be consulted for a definition of decibels, toleration levels, and related phenomena.) The airport will usually provide a guide who can answer specific technical questions, and who might even give a short lecture on noise pollution. It is important that the teacher clearly indicate the reason for the trip so that it will be given proper emphasis. (As usual, the teacher must check on school procedure concerning scheduling of the trip, bus rental or other transportation, written parental permission, lunch facilities, and airport restrictions.)

3. *What Is Sound?* In order to fully understand the problem of noise pollution, students must understand the way in which the ear functions. The teacher can provide copies of a diagram of the internal structure of the ear similar to Figure 4-1, and use an overhead or opaque projector.

Students should understand that sound begins when a vibrating object causes air around it to vibrate. As the vibrations pass from molecule to molecule, they may be intercepted by the ear. *What is actually bombarding the eardrum?* The vibrating air is funneled into the ear by the outer ear or pinna, and then hits the eardrum or tympanic membrane. The vibrations of the membrane cause the hammer (malleus), anvil (incus), and stirrup (stapes) to vibrate in turn. These tiny bones are located in the middle ear. Since the stirrup leads into the inner ear, the vibrations now move

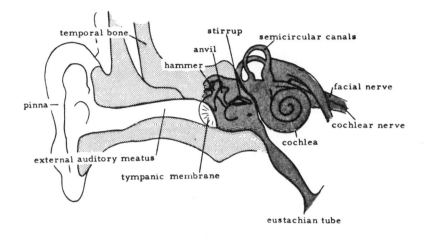

Figure 4-1. Ear

on to the fluid of the inner ear, causing the hairlike projections there to vibrate. These vibrations send impulses along the acoustic nerve to the brain for interpretation. *Is there any point at which extreme or intense noise can cause problems?* Students may have read about the medical concern about potential deafness due to listening to very loud music. The teacher can here explain the phenomenon known as soft pedalling by which the tympanic membrane compensates for very loud vibrations by vibrating less. This protects the inner ear, but eventually the membrane may become unable to vibrate fully at normal sound levels, causing deafness. *What happens if very severe vibrations hit the eardrum?* Eardrum ruptures due to loud explosions can be introduced. Thickening of the membrane due to the formation of the scar tissue can be mentioned. *Is the eardrum the only structure that is susceptible to damage?*

Students will be interested to note that in September, 1968, several reports on the effects of rock music on the ears of guinea pigs were released. Various scientists recorded rock music in

several discotheques, and then played it back to an audience of
guinea pigs. After some ninety hours of intermittent exposure to
the music, the cells of the cochlea were photographed. They had
collapsed and shriveled up like prunes.

4. *Laboratory Activity.* A number of laboratory experiments can be used to study the nature of the functioning of the
ear. The Weber Test can be performed in the laboratory to test for
soft pedalling. Have students work in pairs in an average room, not
a completely quiet one. The observer should place the handle of a
vibrating tuning fork against the center of the subject's forehead.
In normal hearing, the subject will be aware of the sound at the
midline of the head. If one ear is soft pedalling, as in the case of
someone with middle ear deafness, the sound will be heard in the
defective ear, since the normal ear will "soft pedal." This will also
be observed in cases where the subject may have been seated near
a blasting speaker or amplifier within the past few days. (To
simulate middle ear deafness one ear can be plugged with cotton.)

If possible, the teacher should borrow one or several sound
survey meters. These may be available from manufacturers, factories which monitor sound within their premises, or citizens groups
organized to fight excess noise. Since these are not expensive, they
might be included in the school budget. They can be used by
students to randomly measure sound levels. They may also be part
of a more elaborate study organized and executed by the students
themselves. Here, the students may like to bring in recordings of
"noises in the home" and test the sound levels involved.

Interested students, perhaps those considering a future in
medicine, might be interested in researching the work on noise
pollution and its relationship to arteriosclerotic heart disease and
vasoconstriction.

What Can You Do?

1. Do not play your radio, stereo, or television set too
   loudly.
2. Do not sit too closely to a radio or television set that is
   turned on.
3. If you or your parents work in a very noisy atmosphere,
   take precautions to protect your ears from loud noises

or vibrations of a continuous nature. Ear plugs might prove helpful to you in such a situation.

4. Visit your local airport to observe the methods that are used to reduce jet noise and protect the workers from ear damage.

5. Fight for quiet. If there is a manufacturing plant, airport, or other enterprise in your neighborhood that makes excessive noise, form a citizens group and try to reduce or completely eliminate this noise.

6. Have your parents support legislation designed to cut down on noises of various sorts, from that of airports to that of car horns.

Pertinent Facts

1. Noise pollution can cause damage to the ears, heart, lungs, and even to unborn children.

2. A decibel is a unit used to describe the intensity of a sound wave.

3. Sound begins when a vibrating object causes air around it to vibrate.

4. In soft pedalling the tympanic membrane compensates for very severe vibrations by vibrating less.

Possible Quiz

1. Define the term "noise pollution." How is it measured?

2. What factors contribute to noise pollution? How can they be corrected?

3. How does sound carry through the various chambers of the ear?

4. What is meant by soft pedalling?

READINGS

Baker, Bill, and Helen Kotsonis, *Modern Lesson Plans for the Biology Teacher.* West Nyack: Parker Publishing Co., Inc., 1970.

Boughey, Arthur, *Man and the Environment.* New York: The Macmillan Co., 1971.

Holden, J., and Paul Ehrlich, *Global Ecology.* New York: Harcourt, Brace, Jovanovich, Inc., 1971.

Strobbe, Maurice, *Understanding Environmental Pollution.* St. Louis: The C.V. Mosby Co., 1971.

FILMS

"Noise: New Pollutant." 30 minutes, sound, black and white, $7.50. Extension Media, University of California, Berkeley, California.

LESSON 5

Pesticide Pollution

Lesson time: 90 minutes
Laboratory time: 45 minutes

Aim

To conceptualize alternatives to the use of pesticides for the control of insects and other pests from an understanding of their life cycles and characteristics.

Materials

films

Planned Lesson

1. *Insecticides and Insects.* Classroom discussion of pesticides might begin with a general discussion of insecticides, insects, life cycles and characteristics of insects. Students have been exposed to a great deal of publicity warning of the poisoning of our environment with insecticides. They will be able to suggest many of the reasons about which the public is wary; however, they may not have much information about the need for insecticides. The teacher might use the two opposing views to develop an active, interesting discussion which can lead to study in greater depth. Recent news articles can be used to point out the dependence we still have on insecticides. The World Health

Organization reports which suggest that the marked decrease in DDT use in Ceylon has caused a sudden sharp rise in malaria cases, the fact that yearly farm losses due to insects in the U.S. alone average about three billion dollars, and similar news items should help to broaden students' perspectives. This area of study is particularly effective for developing an open-minded attitude in students since so little of the "other side" of the story gets aired.

Before developing a study of insecticide problems, it would be wise to consider the insects themselves. The great range in size and environment of insects should be explored. *What is the highest temperature at which an insect can survive? The lowest? At what altitude ranges are they found?*

Why are insects so successful? Students will usually identify the wide range of environments as one important asset to insects. They may also mention the large numbers of eggs they produce. With some help they will probably also include their ability to fly, their relatively small size, and their protective outer covering. If they are available, large insects, such as grasshoppers, can be examined with hand lenses or binocular microscopes and might then be dissected. *How are they adapted to their way of life?*

In preparation for the study of harmful insects, the teacher might assign the preparation of a list of beneficial and harmful insects and why they are so listed. Students may be surprised to discover that a very small number of insects are harmful to man, animals, or plants. In order to put their study into perspective, however, they might be asked to list the approximate damage insects create in terms of money or other measures. If possible, the library might be asked to add appropriate references to its collection. If these are not available, many standard biology texts also provide such detail. Exterminators, local schools of agriculture, and various pest control agencies will usually supply booklets as well.

2. *How Can We Control Insects?*   The teacher might here begin a presentation dealing with the various means of controlling insects. Rachel Carson's *Silent Spring* would be a worthwhile reading assignment. Beginning historically, discussion can start with the naturally occurring plant products. *Why do television advertisements and other pest control campaigns recommend using*

rotenone or pyrethrin? Because they are naturally occurring, the class should be able to deduce that these would be broken down by natural chemical processes. From this point, discussion can move to the inorganics. Students might speak with older relatives, interview senior citizens, or research old books to learn about the various copper, arsenic, zinc, and other compounds used at the turn of the century. Some reading of labels on the store shelves should provide the class with some of the currently used products. From a careful reading of the product description, the DDT related compounds such as methoxychlor, dieldrin, and chlordane will be listed. *To what group do malathion and parathion belong? Where do the sprays used for mosquitoes belong?*

3. *How Do Insecticides Work?* Research of labels alone should suggest that the various insecticides do not all work the same way. Drawing on their knowledge of the Kreb's cycle, students should be encouraged to consider the effects of enzyme blocks such as arsenic and copper. Recent references will help them to determine the ways in which the others work. Students might write to manufacturers to request information. *Which ones are stomach poisons? Which cause suffocation? What others are there?*

4. *Can We Do Without Pesticides?* By now, students should have facts upon which to base an answer to this question. Stress here should be on an intelligent use of pesticides rather than careless application of them. The "biodegradable" problem should also be included. *What are the safest ways to apply insecticides? Why is spraying unwise?* The unwanted contamination of the environment and its implications can involve much of Miss Carson's material.

5. *Biological Controls. How can the use of pesticides be reduced?* A great deal of current material deals with various uses of biological controls. Irradiating males to induce sterility, chemical lures for trapping, natural predators and other possible means should be considered. The limitations of each should also be considered. *Why must large numbers of sterile males be used if success is to result? What danger is inherent in importing natural enemies?* The class will be aware from their reading that most such techniques are still experimental and include such problems as successfully

raising insects in the laboratory. *Why does the United States help to fund research on insect pests throughout the world? What role might microbes play in future pest control? Is it likely that pesticides will no longer be needed?* The World Health Organization can provide extensive information on insect control throughout the world.

6. *Other Pests.* With the insecticide study as a background, the class will be able to move into rat and other pest control studies smoothly. *What does your community do to control these pests?* Student researchers might contact community departments responsible for dumping, building, and other activities likely to have problems with rodents. They should collect information about the kinds of poisons used and control methods available. If possible, they should investigate the difficulties resulting from the growing resistance rats have to the limited number of poisons which are safe for other animals and therefore the only ones recommended for rodent problems. *How successful are rodent control programs locally? Nationally? On what things does success depend?* The Department of Health, Education, and Welfare as well as local control groups will supply a great deal of information. For international information the World Health Organization is again an excellent source.

7. *Laboratory Activities.* Although laboratory procedures can be developed to show the harm caused by pesticides to organisms, they require the handling of dangerous chemicals, and more importantly, are not humane. Films and slides are available from commercial, as well as public sources, such as Fish and Wildlife Departments, which show the harmful effects more graphically than a laboratory could. It would also be somewhat ironic to teach about the preservation of life by casually destroying it in a laboratory. This point should always be stressed when students plan inhumane projects. Laboratory time can be beneficially used to consider research students have made into pesticides however. After developing lists of pesticides and their ingredients by checking store shelves, they can divide them into categories which might be botanicals (pyrethrin, rotenone), inorganics (arsenic, copper, etc.), DDT relatives (chlordane, methoxychlor, heptachlor, dieldrin, kelthane), phosphorus compounds (dibrom, vapona, malathion, systox), fumigants (paradichlorobenzene, moth balls), and the various petroleum fractions. A number of

books will provide rather complete lists, as will many available pamphlets. Carson's *Silent Spring* and Ehrlich and Ehrlich's *Population, Resources, Environment* are possible sources. This chart can also include information gathered concerning pest control. For example, the compounds used in community control programs should be identified as should those used by exterminators and other private users. *Does your community use the safest possible pesticide? Why has it chosen the ones which are used?* This may lead to a bulletin board display and to the preparation of posters warning about pesticide misuse. A community publicity campaign may be made part of this activity as well. Awareness of current news items should be encouraged. Discussion might include the recent fire ant control program of the United States Department of Agriculture and the controversy it started.

What Can You Do?

1. Warn your parents and friends about the dangers of pesticides and herbicides. Have them cut down on the pesticides they are now using.
2. If your parents have a garden or farm, have them grow only those types of plants that are the most resistant to disease and insects. The same applies for fruits and vegetables. This way you will need less pesticides.
3. If you must use pesticides, be discriminating. Apply them only to those areas affected by the insect or pest.
4. If the town in which you live sprays the trees and plants in your neighborhood, find out what kind of pesticide or insecticide is being used. If toxic or long-lasting chemicals are being used, get them to switch to a less toxic one.
5. Try not to use chlorinated hydrocarbons. They are the most dangerous of the pesticides.

Pertinent Facts

1. Man has never been able to eradicate even a single species of insect.
2. Insects are successful because of their many characteristics which make them adaptable to many environments.

3. Insects, completely uncontrolled by natural or artificial means, would probably destroy all of the vegetation on the earth in one year.
4. Rodents are responsible for the destruction of large amounts of food as well as for spread of disease and other threats to mankind.
5. Use of pesticides is essential for control of harmful organisms today, but they must be used wisely and with caution.

Possible Quiz

1. Give four characteristics of insects which help to make them successful and indicate why each is important.
2. Of the 670,000–250,000 insect species, about 900 are harmful. Identify ten of these and indicate why they are harmful.
3. Discuss some of the biological controls now being investigated and tested.
4. Indicate three different ways in which a pesticide might work and give an example of a commercial product for each.
5. Discuss any local community control project, giving materials used and procedure followed. Compare disadvantages and advantages.

READINGS

Borgstrom, G., *The Hungry Planet.* New York: Collier, 1965.

de Bach, Paul, ed., *Biological Control of Insects, Pests, and Weeds.* New York: Rheinhold, 1965.

Hoffman, C.H., and L.S. Henderson, *Protecting our Food, Yearbook of Agriculture,* "The Fight Against Insects," Chapter 3, U.S. Government Printing Office, 1966.

Knipling, E.F., "The Eradication of the Screw-Worm Fly," *Scientific American,* Vol, 203, No. 54, 1960.

Rudd, R., *Pesticides and the Living Landscape.* Madison, Wisconsin: University of Wisconsin Press, 1964.

FILMS

"Silent Spring of Rachel Carson." 54 minutes, sound, black and white. Indiana University, A-V Center, Bloomington, Indiana 47401.

"A Plague on Your Children." 72 minutes, sound, black and white. British Broadcasting Corporation. Available from: Peter M. Roebeck and Company, 230 Park Avenue, New York, N.Y. 10017.

LESSON 6

Pollution and
Food Additives

Lesson time: 45 minutes
Laboratory time: 45-90 minutes

Aim

To explore the uses of food additives, the reasons for their use, and the harmful effects they can produce in human tissue; and to determine in the laboratory which common foods have additives in them.

Materials

funnels	glass rods
pipettes	Erlenmeyer flasks
beakers	micropipettes
steam bath	filter paper (Whatman No. 3MM, 7" x 9")
small aquarium	cotton
oranges	chloroform
light mineral oil	ethyl ether
acetone	distilled or deionized water
Citrus Red No. 2	Oil Red XO*

---

*These may be obtained free of charge—see Section 5 of Planned Lesson.

Planned Lesson

1. *Is Our Food Safe?*   The teacher will want to stress the need for safe food for well-being and general good health, together with the related problem of the need for a safety control. Students should be asked to give examples of ways in which the consumer may suffer from "unsafe" foods. *What would a safe food be?*

The teacher can begin by referring to the occasional news stories of contamination, such as glass in foods, bugs baked into loaves of bread, or similar incidents. Three main problems can then be identified: poisons in food (botulism), disease infestation (salmonella), and foreign substances which can cause such injuries as choking, nausea, and internal damage. This can logically lead to a discussion of means to protect the consumer. *Is one federal set of rules better than individual local or state control? What is the name of the federal agency involved? Does your state and/or town also have food laws? Why might these be necessary?*

At this point the teacher can include a discussion of the so-called "incidental" additives. Student discussion should center around the residues which enter our foods as they are growing or when they are processed. These might include residues of pesticides, drugs, cleaning materials, and other chemicals. *How do these contaminate food? Where do they come from? How do they affect us?*

2. *How Can the Consumer Find Out About a Product?*   Students should be familiarized with the various consumer safeguards, including labeling. A student assignment might be to ask students to read the labels on ten different packages and list the kinds of information given, such as weight, contents, and grade. Some students can be asked to do research to determine what the laws require to be on a label. *Does your city have laws concerning labeling? What standards do federal laws set for foods? Is all mayonnaise the same? Why?* The teacher should stress that federal laws only govern interstate commerce. Since standards for interstate sales are uniform, all products identified by the same name, i.e. mayonnaise, must meet minimum standards for that product.

3. *What Are "Additives?" Why Use Them?*   Students have

no doubt heard about or read news stories concerning various food additives, and should be able to give a basic definition. The teacher can make a list of these student suggestions and place it on the chalkboard. The list will probably include the various preservatives such as those found listed on cereal labels; cyclamates; saccharin and other artificial sweeteners; vitamins as in milk and cereals; various minerals; and artificial coloring. Students may have to be reminded that additives are not just the "foreign" substances, but also such things as salt, sugar, and spices.

A discussion based on this list can bring out the many benefits of additives: improved flavor, longer lasting breads, less calories, better nutritional value, substitution for medically dangerous foods (as in diabetes), and greater aesthetic appeal.

4. *Who Controls the Use of Additives?* The teacher can continue the concept of the FDA and federal laws and their control of additive use. The issue of the use of cyclamates in foods can be used as the focal point of the discussion. The testing programs used, the idea of an approved list of additives, and outside research should be included.

What is a "safe" additive? The teacher can use the cyclamates as an example of an additive that was restricted as a result of research in which large amounts were given to rats; the rats subsequently developed cancer. Of course, no valid conclusions can be drawn in the high school classroom, but the teacher can stimulate the use of the scientific method as the basis of student thinking. *Would the results of research on rats or mice apply to man? What limitations would exist?* Scientific thought might again be stressed when students consider mass use of "fad" substances. *Do you think out your purchases or buy what everyone else is buying? Do you know what additives are in the foods you eat? Are these additives necessary for all people?*

Students can obtain copies of the FDA "Additives in Our Food," which is part of the Life Protection Series. With this and other sources, they can list the requirements additives must meet in order to be approved for use.

5. *How Can You Test for Additives in Your Laboratory?* The teacher can use several excellent laboratory exercises which have been developed for the FDA for testing for additives.

These are valuable because they make use of a variety of laboratory techniques as well as illustrating possible tests for additives.

Specific equipment needed for this activity includes:

2 funnels, 125mm	6 glass rods
2 pipettes, 25 ml	2 Erlenmeyer flasks, 125 ml
2 beakers, 100 ml	1 micropipette
1 steam bath	1 funnel support
2 sheets Whatman	
No. 3MM filter paper,	1 aquarium
7" x 9"	oranges (3 stamped color added, 3 not stamped)
cotton	
chloroform, 300 ml	ethyl ether, 95 ml
light mineral oil, 5 grams	distilled or deionized water,
acetone, 200 ml	100 ml
Citrus Red No. 2, 1-(2,5-	Oil Red XO (1-xylyazo-2-
dimethoxphenylazo)-2	napthol), approximately 0.1
napthol, approximately	gm
0.1 gm	

Small quantities of Citrus Red No. 2 and Oil Red XO may be obtained free of charge if requested on your official school stationery, by writing to: Mr. Raymond V. Leary, Product Manager, National Aniline Division, Allied Chemical Corporation, 40 Rector Street, New York, New York 10006.

Students may be asked to volunteer for the advance preparations that are necessary. The sheet of filter paper must be placed on a flat surface so that the 9" dimension is vertical, and the 7" dimension is horizontal. Using a soft lead pencil, draw a horizontal line across the sheet 1 inch from the bottom edge. Then mark off on the line three 1½" segments, approximately ½" apart. The 1½ inch segments should be labeled as follows: First sheet: (1.) Citrus Red No. 2; (2.) "color added" oranges; (3.) Oil Red XO; Second sheet: (1.) Citrus Red No. 2; (2.) oranges not stamped "color added"; (3.) Oil Red XO.

A solution of mineral oil in ethyl ether should be prepared by dissolving 5 grams of the oil in 95ml of ether. Stir until thoroughly mixed. Transfer to the 100ml graduated cylinder. Immerse one rolled sheet of paper in the mineral oil solution for a few minutes. Remove and dry by suspending it in air. Treat the second sheet in the same way. (*Note:* ether is highly flammable and should be kept away from open flames or electric heating elements.)

Prepare a mixture of 130ml of acetone and 70ml of distilled water. Stir until mixed and store until ready for use in a glass-stoppered bottle.

Place a small piece of cotton in the bottom of a 125ml filtering funnel supported on a stand. Position three glass rods in the funnel in such a manner that they will support an orange so that it will not touch the sides of the funnel. Prepare standard solutions of the two dyes as follows: dissolve 10mg of Citrus Red No. 2 in 50ml of chloroform. Store in a glass-stoppered bottle away from light. Dissolve 10mg of Oil Red XO in 50ml of chloroform. Store in a labeled glass-stoppered bottle away from light.

During the laboratory period itself, the following procedures should be followed:

a. Set water to boil if steam bath is not available (for step d).

b. Place a 125ml Erlenmeyer flask beneath the funnel and support an orange on the glass rods. Wash the color off a "color added" orange by spraying it with 25ml of chloroform in the form of a fine stream from a pipette. (Use rubber tubing on the end of the pipette; a medicine dropper can also be used in place of the pipette.) Surface oils, waxes, and natural pigments as well as the artificial color will be washed off.

c. Repeat step b with two more of the "color added" oranges, combining the washings in the same flask.

d. Transfer a portion of the solution of these washings to a 100ml beaker. Allow the solution in the beaker to evaporate by placing the beaker in a steam bath in a fume hood, or over a suitable container of hot water if a steam bath is not available. *Note:* it is important to use a fume hood since the evaporating fumes are irritating and can be harmful. When the solvent has evaporated, add another small portion of the solution. (Remember that the fumes are those of chloroform and must be treated with care.) Continue the evaporation until all the solution has been transferred and all solvent has evaporated.

e. Using another 125ml flask, and a clean funnel, glass rods, and so forth, repeat steps b, c, and d, using the unstamped oranges. While the evaporating process is taking place, students can go on to step f.

f. Pour the prepared acetone solution into the bottom of the aquarium. Transfer a 50 microliter portion (approximate) of each of the prepared solutions of Citrus Red No. 2 and Oil Red XO to the marked sheets of filter paper, prepared earlier. This can be done by dipping a pointed capillary tube or melting point tube into the solutions and drawing the liquid in a band along the appropriate 1½" lines on the filter paper. Allow the chloroform to evaporate from the paper for about 5 seconds, and retrace the line two more times in the same manner. Allow drying between applications. Finally, suspend the papers in air to dry.

g. Allow the beakers to cool after removing them from the steam bath. Dissolve the residue in each beaker in 3ml of chloroform. Transfer a 50 microliter portion of the "color added" extract to the first sheet of prepared filter paper in the same manner you used with the authentic dye solutions; repeat with the second sheet, using the extract from the uncolored oranges.

h. Both sheets should be lowered into the aquarium so that the 9" dimension is vertical, and suspended so that the bottom edge of the paper is immersed about ¼" into the solvent. The papers should not touch each other or the tank. The tank should then be covered with a plate of glass and allowed to stand for approximately one hour.

i. After an hour, the sheets should be removed and dried as before. The distance between the colors should be measured and compared. The natural coloring materials will not move up the paper. A discussion of the experiment should follow. *What were the results? How does the chromatography method work? If a spot was*

*found which traveled a distance different from either
known color, what might that indicate?*

Other useful and interesting experiments students can perform may be found in the FDA pamphlets, "Identity of Synthetic
Colors in Foods," and "Rapid Identity of Margarine and Butter."

What Can You Do?

1. Grow your own fruits and vegetables. This will limit the
   use of preservatives in your food.
2. Eat more fresh fruits and vegetables.
3. Try to buy more fruits and vegetables that have been
   grown "organically."

Pertinent Facts

1. Foods are considered "safe" if they are free from
   contaminants which can cause poisoning, disease, or
   internal injury.
2. The Food and Drug Administration has the responsibility for controlling the quality of all foods manufactured or sold in interstate commerce.
3. Federal laws control the labeling, standards, and additives which are used by the food industry.
4. Additives are added to foods to improve them in some
   way.
5. The individual consumer should always be aware of the
   additives in the foods he uses.

Possible Quiz

1. What kinds of contaminants may be found in foods?
   Why are they dangerous?
2. Why are federal laws needed for food control? Why are
   state and local laws needed?
3. What are five kinds of information you would expect to
   find on a label? Why are labeling laws important?
4. What is a food additive? Why are food additives useful?

5. List five specific additives used and give the reasons for their use.

READINGS

Food and Drug Administration, "Additives in Our Food." Washington, D.C.: United States Government Printing Office, 1967.

Food and Drug Administration, "Identity of Synthetic Colors in Food," "Rapid Identity of Margarine and Butter," and "Identity of Artificial Color on Oranges." Washington, D.C.: United States Government Printing Office, 1967.

Stare, Frederick, "The Balance Is All in Their Favor." *Look Magazine,* February, 1970.

FILMS

"A Reason for Confidence." 28 minutes, sound, color, free. National Medical Audiovisual Center, Annex, Chamblee, Georgia 30005. Attention: Distribution.

"The Health Fraud Racket." 28 minutes, sound, black and white, free. National Medical Audiovisual Center, Annex.

Overhead projection materials to be used in conjunction with the FDA materials may be obtained from: DCA Educational Products, Inc. 4865 Stenton Avenue, Philadelphia, Pa. 19144.

LESSON 7

Radioactivity
and Pollution

Lesson time: 90 minutes
Laboratory time: 90 minutes

Aim

To trace the effects of radiation on a living plant in the laboratory through the use of radioisotopes and Geiger counters, and to hypothesize the larger implications of radiation for all forms of life.

Materials

Geiger counter	dosimeter
film badges	coleus plant
uranium nitrate solution	photographic hypo
X-ray film	

Planned Lesson

1. *Radiation.* In preparation for a study of the effects of radiation on man and his environment, some background material should be presented. This might include introductory material on Henri Becquerel and Pierre and Marie Curie. Short oral reports or

written papers could be assigned in advance or film strips or other audio-visuals could be used. Other films or film strips might follow providing a basis upon which to study radiation. This material should include some understanding of alpha, beta, and gamma rays, and X rays. *Why are these called ionizing radiation?* It might also be necessary to briefly review atomic structure. The presence of protons and neutrons in the nucleus and electrons moving in orbits around it and the balance between positive (protons) particles and negative (electrons) particles should be noted. The teacher can then go on to explain bonding and the subsequent change in the number of electrons. This then leads directly to an explanation of ionization. It would be valuable to carry this one step further to a discussion of electrolytes. *Why does a solution which contains ions conduct electricity? Why do we call intravenous solutions which replace various body substances electrolytes?*

After such a review the class might move into a deeper study of radiation. It is important that the class consider the differences in the characteristics of the radiations. Most elementary physics or general science texts can provide material for student researchers. They should be able to distinguish between alpha particles (hydrogen nuclei), beta particles (electrons) and gamma rays. They should also realize that alpha particles can penetrate soft tissue but can be stopped by most materials including our skin or a thin sheet of paper. Beta particles, on the other hand, need a cinder block shield or they will penetrate into skin. Gamma rays are most dangerous since they can penetrate deep into matter and we require more than clothing or cinder blocks to protect us. *What are some sources of each type of radiation?*

2. *How Is Radiation Measured?*   Students should determine the definition for roentgen (and perhaps some information about Roentgen) and for rem. They might also check into local Civil Defense sources for additional information on the levels of roentgen equivalents man (rem) which cause illness and death. They should understand that the rem is more significant biologically since it offers some standardized means of comparison.

3. *Half Life.*   In order to understand the problems involved with radioactive materials, the class should know about half life. The teacher must again emphasize that ionizing radiation is so named because it knocks electrons out of atoms, thus causing

ionization. This ionization is the actual agent which causes biological changes. *How long does this reactivity (ionization) last?* The length of time required for half the atoms to disintegrate, or half life, can be identified for various substances. *Why is a substance like Iodine–131 (half life 8 days) used to treat disease rather than Cesium–137? Why are biologists concerned about the continued presence of Strontium 90 in the environment?* Here there should be the realization the iodine's short half life provides radiation for a short time, but is soon harmless, while strontium and cesium have very long half lives. Interested students might report on carbon–14 dating.

4. *Sources of Radiation.* A class prepared chart can include: various sources of natural radiation contributing to background radiation such as cosmic rays; the various naturally occurring radioactive elements; and levels of each which are considered safe. Sources would also include nuclear power plants, testing of nuclear weapons, manufacturing processes, use of X-rays, and various other uses of radioactive materials in medical treatment. A number of interesting reports could be generated from this assignment including the specific medical uses of radioactive materials, the uses of irradiation in the preservation of food, and the many uses for radioactive tracers and materials in biological research.

5. *Problems of Radiation Pollution.* From their study of acceptable levels of radiation, students have already focused on the chief concern of environmentalists involving radiation. The term "fallout" is probably familiar, but its definition as radioactive particles should be re-emphasized. *Why is fallout of such concern?* The dangers of fallout should be considered in some detail. Its ability to seriously burn and to provide large doses of whole-body irradiation is sometimes underestimated because it is "dust." How serious the actual effects of such exposure are has been studied only under limited conditions and so no absolutes can be given. Many of the elements which become radioactive and are part of fallout are absorbed readily by plants and so enter the food chains. It is also important for students to consider and understand the importance of global control of nuclear testing which can be included in a discussion of fallout.

Other important radiation problems are related to atomic

reactors. The disposal of wastes from reactors is a serious problem recently receiving more and more publicity. Nuclear reactors are devices in which controlled fission of radioactive material produces new radioactive substances and energy. The energy is released as heat, captured by water circulating in the reactor which becomes steam, and is used as steam to drive turbines to produce electricity. The new radioactive substances must be disposed of and this is a problem. *What possible ways are there to dispose of this material? What problems are involved?* Burying of the material, sealing it in special containers, and sinking it should be considered as to feasibility and dangers. If the group is interested, it might be worthwhile to explore in some detail the operation of various types of reactors. Most elementary physics books deal with them as do many specialized textbooks and handbooks. Information is available from research laboratories such as Brookhaven National Laboratories, Brookhaven, Long Island, N.Y., or the many other accelerator facilities throughout the country. *What other pollution problem do you see as likely to result from reactors?*

Because water is taken from nearby bodies of water and usually is returned to that source somewhat warmer than when it was removed, there is also a problem of thermal pollution. Generally, nuclear plant administrators insist that they do not contribute to thermal pollution, but many concerned citizens have charged that the plants generally do raise the temperature of the water at least 1°C. Calling on their earlier study of thermal pollution, students will remember that enzymatic functions are carefully regulated in biological systems and that temperature is one of the major factors involved. Even more significant is that less oxygen can dissolve in the water as its temperature increases. This is critical since oxygen is not very soluble in water under ideal conditions. As conditions become adverse, the amount of oxygen dissolved becomes critically low. *Would such water be considered polluted?* As our earlier definition (Lesson 1—Water Pollution) suggests, the amount of available oxygen is the criterion by which microbiologists measure water pollution.

Overexposure to sources of radiation is not limited to explosions of nuclear weapons as in Hiroshima and Nagasaki. *What situations could cause such exposure? Why does an X-ray tech-*

nician, dentist, or other operator always wear a protective lead apron, stand behind a shield or leave the room? A number of industrial and medical situations could be noted, although it should be pointed out that radiation treatment involves highly sophisticated machines which can be adjusted so that tissue above and below the target area will be completely unharmed while the target cells are destroyed. Articles in medical journals, biological abstracts, and other similar sources can be used by those interested to learn about accidents which have occurred and the results of them.

6. *Effects of Exposure to Radiation.* Because we are always exposed to background radiation, we receive an average of about ten roentgens of nuclear radiation in a lifetime from this source. We also receive small amounts from medical and dental X rays, certain electrical equipment, the soil, rocks, and even from luminous watch dials. Generally, students tend to think of the harmful results of overdoses of radiation such as radiation sickness and tissue burns. They should be encouraged to seek information on the beneficial effects ranging from the already mentioned treatment for abnormal cell growth to the use of tracer substances to determine the physiological behavior of some organs to sterilization of equipment as well as foods. This means of preservation of food could provide an interesting report topic as could the whole field of agriculture research with radiation. The World Health Organization might be contacted for information concerning its many research teams throughout the world, some of which use radioactive wire, for example, to glue onto insects so that they can be located with Geiger counters. Major industries which require constant monitoring of thicknesses, joints, and similar characteristics of their products may be using radiation sensors. If possible, a field trip to such a plant should be arranged. Some reading and investigating will provide students with a surprisingly long and varied list of uses. They should be asked to determine in each case an explanation of the process involved.

Specifically, they should then be able to consider how the radiation actually affects the organism or object exposed to it. This will also provide a thorough review of the lesson. As suggested in the introduction, a review of the nature of ions and ionization would be very valuable in discussing the effects on living things. Their research of the definition of the roentgen can be called into play here. They know that this measure involves the number of ions produced in a unit volume of air. They also know that ions are charged particles which can be the vehicle for electron movement and are likely to combine with other ions if possible. They should be able to conclude that this can seriously alter the delicate balance in the cell which normally would not have produced these ions in this quantity at this time.

This balance should be spelled out to include the all-important DNA. The lesson might be particularly valuable immediately following the study of chromosomes and their control of cellular metabolism. Readings such as excerpts from Ehrlich and the *Environmental Handbook* (see bibliography) should be used to acquaint students with the still raging controversy of the effects of radiation on us and on future generations. *Does excess radiation cause cancer, birth defects, stillbirths?* This can be carried through to the industrial uses of radiation as well. *In industry how are workers protected from exposure to radiation? Does the radioactivity affect the product itself? When fruit is exposed to radiation so that bacteria on its surface can be destroyed, are the tissues of the fruit injured? Explain.*

7. *Laboratory Activities.*   Teams of students can monitor the classroom and use sources of alpha and beta radiation as they learn to operate detection devices.

If the school does not have Geiger counters and the somewhat more elaborate scalers, the local Civil Defense unit will usually be willing to lend some and will frequently also provide a lecturer to demonstrate their use. They may also include dosimeters, film badges, and other detectors. The students can use physics and general science texts to read about the operation of the Geiger counter and its sensitive Geiger-Muller tube. They should be warned to handle all equipment gently. The various scalers, although apparently more complex, are really just desk models with the same operating principles.

Manufacturers generally provide plastic encased alpha and beta sources which can be used. Although there is no danger in using weak radioisotopes in the school laboratory if proper precautions are taken, the teacher would be wise to check for any special school regulations. Uranium nitrate is a commonly used and easily obtained isotope. It can be used in a number of different types of experiments. Frequently when students have been introduced to general techniques they will devise some interesting experiments of their own. Plants are the recommended subjects for study since animal experiments will require that animals be sacrificed and various organs tested separately.

If no Geiger counters are available, students can prepare a solution of uranium nitrate and stand the stem of a plant, such as a geranium or coleus, in it for several hours. They should then place a leaf from the experimental plant on an unopened package of X-ray film. As a control, a similar leaf from an untreated plant should also be on the film. A weight, such as several books, should be used to hold the leaves flat. The setup should be stored in a closet or other dark place for two weeks. After this time, they may have a local hospital or technician develop the plate (also an excellent opportunity for a group trip to visit such facilities) or they may use plain household vinegar to wash the unwrapped plate and then place it in photographic hypo for fifteen to twenty minutes. A glass or enamel pan should be used for the hypo which can be bought at most department stores or camera shops. Because it is not light sensitive, the film may be developed in the normal classroom situation.

The same solution can be used to measure the rate of movement of water through a plant. Two plants of the same type and about the same size should be kept side by side for several days and watered the same measured amount at the same time. These should then be used as experimental and control plants. One being watered as usual, the other receiving the same amount but of uranium nitrate solution. Using a Geiger counter, the class can trace the passage of the radioisotope solution. *Why should you determine the background radiation count first? Why should you use a control?*

There are a great many other possible laboratory procedures which can be developed using this basic technique. The Atomic Energy Commission provides some isotopes for high school use

through distribution centers. The Washington, D.C. Office of the
AEC (Washington, D.C. 20025) can supply more information on
this program and on its various publications regarding use, precautions, and other activities.

What Can You Do?

1. Have your parents press for and support legislation
   designed to eliminate the dangers of radiation leakage
   from such items as color television sets and radar ovens.
2. If your parents have just bought a color television set,
   have the man that installs it go over it with a Geiger
   counter to insure that it is not giving off excessive
   radioactivity. The same should apply if your parents
   have just purchased a radar oven or other similar device.
3. Do not sit too closely to a color television set that is in
   operation. Sit at least six to eight feet away from it.
4. Visit a local power plant and learn firsthand the precautions taken to insure that no leakage of radioactive
   materials occurs.

Pertinent Facts

1. Alpha particles can be stopped by many materials,
   including skin.
2. Beta particles require a cinder block shield to prevent
   their penetrating the skin.
3. Gamma rays are the most deeply penetrating rays.
4. Ionizing radiation knocks electrons out of atoms, thus
   causing ionization.
5. Half life is the length of time required for half the atoms
   in a sample of radioactive material to disintegrate.

Possible Quiz

1. What is the nature of the three types of radiation? What
   shielding is needed to protect against each of them?

2. Identify some of the forms of pollution caused by nuclear power plants. Why is each of concern to us?
3. What are some important beneficial uses of radiation? Explain three in some detail.
4. What kinds of changes occur in a cell which has been exposed to high levels of radiation?
5. What kinds of devices can be used to detect the presence of radiation? Explain how to use any one of these.

READINGS

Blatz, Hanson, *Introduction to Radiological Health.* New York: McGraw-Hill, 1964.

Comar, C.L., *Radioisotopes in Biology and Agriculture.* New York: McGraw-Hill, 1955.

Eisenbud, Merrill, *Environmental Radioactivity.* New York: McGraw-Hill, 1963.

Hollaender, A., ed., *Radiation Biology.* New York: McGraw-Hill, 1954-1956, 3 volumes.

Schenberg, S. and J. Harley, *Laboratory Experiments with Radioisotopes for High School Science Teachers.* Washington, D.C.: Superintendent of Documents, U.S. Government Printing Office, 1957.

FILMS

"Radiological Defense." 27 minutes, sound, color, $1.15. Indiana University, A-V Department, Bloomington, Indiana.

"Radiotherapy: High Dosage Treatment." 17 minutes, sound, black and white, $2.90. Indiana University.

Conservation
and the
Environment

UNIT 2

LESSON 8

Land Conservation

Lesson time: 45 minutes
Laboratory time: 90 minutes

Aim

To describe the interrelationships between living creatures and the land they occupy using a small block of earth as a representation of a land area in microcosm, and emphasizing wise and protective use of the land by man.

Materials

soil samples
glass slides
microscopes
methylene blue

Planned Lesson

1. *How Do We Use and Abuse Land?* Perhaps students can develop lists of uses as an out-of-class activity. The lists will probably include raising food, living space, forests, recreational facilities. Many abuses can be gathered from other lessons such as the ones concerning pesticides, radioactive fallout, and pollutants from water. Other aspects to be considered: erosion caused by removing trees and plants, increased paving of land, increased

73

building of dwellings, and inundation of land due to dam building. The Aswan Dam project can be used as an example of a man-made change which has altered land use. A great deal of information concerning the project is available to students in newspaper and magazine articles.

As a field and laboratory experience the class might be asked to collect soil samples and examine them carefully. A good sized sample would be a block ten to fourteen inches in each dimension. Students should carefully dig such a block of dirt out and gently place it in a cardboard box so that it can be transferred to the laboratory for study. Small groups might work together to describe color, texture, moisture, and odor of the soil and then, after careful and gentle examination, to identify any organisms present. They should search for small eggs as well as for insects, earthworms, and other common soil creatures. To complete the study they can prepare a simple slide to search for microscopic organisms and may even want to use a simple dye to help them. Methylene blue will work well here. *What benefits do these organisms derive from living in the soil? Do they help the soil? How?*

2. *Erosion.* If such a site is available, it will be valuable to have the class observe an excavation which has exposed several layers of the soil profile. *What differences can you see? What makes the topsoil different from the subsoil? Why is topsoil important?* These questions can lead into the need to protect the topsoil and to the various means by which it is eroded. Deforestation, poor irrigation practices, and overgrazing should be dealt with as prime factors caused by man.

Interesting research reports can be developed on the origin of some of the great deserts, as the Sahara, to illustrate the roles played by man in the loss of topsoil and the ultimate loss of available land.

A class project or field trip can involve observation of erosion. This need not be a large area but may be a slope in a nearby park or some area around the school. *How can you help prevent erosion?* Here discussion can center around the importance of roots holding soil particles in place. The group can plant ground cover such as pachysandra or, for steep slopes, a quick growing low maintenance crown vetch. *What procedures might be needed if the slope is badly eroded?* Here discussion could include the use of boards, logs, or other braces to hold soil in place until plants have established themselves.

How is topsoil made? Using the laboratory study of organisms in soil and some consideration of the decay of plant material, the production of topsoil can be discussed. It is important to note that it requires many years to produce one inch of topsoil (which can be washed or blown away in minutes if not anchored). The drought in the 1930's which produced the "Dust Bowl" can be introduced here as can the more recent March-April 1971 drought in the Southwest which was said to have removed topsoil that was produced over many decades.

Why is conservation of land so hard to accomplish in underdeveloped countries? The interrelations between lack of food, overgrazing, and deforestation should be explored here.

What problems do developed countries face? A great many public announcements are devoted to road building because it is covering land. Students need to consider the implications of this paving. *What land uses does road building eliminate?* These should include building of houses, planting of food, and recreation.

The lesson can be consolidated by reviewing the study of soil organisms and expanding the concepts to include the entire chain of life dependent on the soil, from smallest microorganisms to man. The class should be able to trace the food chain they might expect to find on a given piece of land.

3. *Parks and Recreation.* The class can consider the use of land for parks and recreation. Originally established as areas for human enjoyment and vacationing, national parks, for example, are now greatly concerned with the conservation of plants and animals as well as with the land itself. A number of articles in *National Wildlife, Time,* and other magazines have stressed the serious problems created when over two million people a season visit a park such as Yellowstone National Park.

Why are parks important? Students might list the photosynthetic production of oxygen on which we depend, but many will think in terms of the psychological values and the need for relaxation and recreation in a setting of natural beauty. It should be noted that as population increase causes the loss of forests and other underdeveloped lands, the establishment of parks becomes more important. Students might write to the Parks Department of New York City, Philadelphia, or other large cities for information on the provisions for parks and planting in their city plans and zoning laws. Many have very specific requirements for plazas, miniparks, and plantings. The material in the lesson on waste disposal might suggest to the students the possibility of using landfill sites, unsafe for building, as parks. They might be interested in the parks built in many European cities on top of piles of the rubble of buildings destroyed in World War II.

What Can You Do?

1. With your supervision, students might develop a vacant lot into a minipark, with proper permission from owner or city, school, and parents, of course. Here they could develop erosion preventive plantings, improve the area, and generally become involved in a community project. They would need to plan, obtain funds and the donations of materials and labor, and then arrange for maintenance. (This could also be done on school property.)
2. Have your parents support the strengthening of planning laws.
3. Help beautify your neighborhood. Organize committees to set up litter baskets; make war on signs; have your neighbors clean up and maintain their gardens and property.

Pertinent Facts

1. We use land as a source of food, for recreation, and living space. We abuse it by adding many foreign chemicals to it, paving over it, overgrazing it, or otherwise interfering with its normal life cycle.
2. A great many organisms live in the soil aerating it, adding to its organic matter, or helping it to break down.

3. The soil is composed of several different layers which constitute the soil profile. These layers include topsoil, subsoil, and bedrock.
4. Erosion causes the loss of valuable topsoil which will take years to be replaced.
5. Increased population puts increased demand on land for agriculture, roads, recreation, and building. Current concern reflects the need for balanced land use.

Possible Quiz

1. What are some of the ill effects of the thoughtless use of land?
2. What organisms might be found in soil? What functions do they perform?
3. How is topsoil made? Why is the loss of topsoil through erosion so significant and dangerous?
4. What are some important problems related to land conservation in underdeveloped countries? Developed countries?
5. How can the public influence land use? Should the public try to influence land use discussions?

READINGS

Cornell Rural School Leaflet, *Conservation: A Handbook for Teachers.* Vol. 45:1, September, 1951.

Jarrett, Henry, ed., *Environmental Quality in a Growing Environment.* Baltimore: Johns-Hopkins Press, 1966.

Udall, Stewart L., *1976, Agenda for Tomorrow.* New York: Harcourt, Brace, and World, Inc., 1968.

FILMS

"Bulldozed America." 25 minutes, sound, black and white, $5.00. University of Michigan, A-V Department, 416 Fourth Street, Ann Arbor, Michigan 48103.

"County Agricultural Agent." Sound, color, Venard Organization, 702
    South Adams Street, Peoria, Illinois.

"Life of the Soil." Sound, color, free, National Fertilizer Association, 616
    Continental Building, Washington D.C. 20005.

"Raindrops and Soil Erosion." Sound, color. U.S. Department of Agriculture,
    Washington, D.C. 20025.

LESSON 9

Plant Conservation

Lesson time: 45 minutes
Laboratory time: 45 minutes

Aim

To discover the importance of a healthy environment and adequate sunlight, water and minerals to plant growth in experiments where plants are deprived of these elements; and to develop methods of arresting such problems in the environment.

Materials

films
nutrient solutions
   lacking nitrate,
   sulphate or phosphate

potted geranium plants
field gathered
   polluted water

Planned Lesson

To introduce this topic the teacher should review the various aspects of the balance of nature.

1. *What Conditions Are Important in the Survival of a Plant?* A list will develop which will include water, minerals, and sunlight. This should be expanded so that all the ramifications of each of these are brought out. Considering water, the class should

review the functions of roots and root hairs. This will naturally lead to the role of roots as anchors for both the plant and for soil particles. (This erosion-preventing role can be reviewed from lesson 8.) The water cycle, water pollution, water as a solvent, the functions of xylem and phloem, and even cell permeability can be discussed if the teacher chooses.

The importance of minerals can be demonstrated by growing plants in nutrient solutions which lack nitrate, sulphate or phosphate. The growing of plants in water nutrient solutions is called hydroponics. *Why is water used in place of soil?* Seeds should be germinated in a petri dish or moist blotting paper.

After two weeks (germination should be begun in advance), roots will have developed sufficiently and the seedlings can be used. Each seedling will need to be supported over a container of distilled water. A number of suitable techniques work well: a series of test tubes, each containing a single seedling supported by a one-hole rubber stopper; a series of beakers each containing a single seedling supported by aluminum foil stretched across the top of the beaker, in which a suitable hole has been punched (or a piece of cheesecloth similarly prepared); or glass jars, glasses, or paper cups. Students will no doubt offer suggestions of their own.

The control seedlings should be placed in solutions which contain all essential minerals for normal growth. Although many different solutions may be used, only two have been included here.

Knop's Solution (weigh out the following and dissolve in 1 liter of distilled water):

$FePO_4$ . . . . trace
KNO_3 . . . . 0.2 gm
$MgSO_4 \bullet 7H_2O$ . . . . 0.2 gm
KH_2PO_4 . . . . 0.2 gm
$Ca(NO_3)_2 \bullet 4H_2O$ . . . . 0.8 gm

Haas and Reed's A to Z Solution (includes trace elements). Weigh out the following and dissolve in 1 liter of distilled water:

H_3BO_3 . . . . 0.6 gm
$MnCl_2 \bullet 4H_2O$ . . . . 0.4 gm
$ZnSO_4$ . . . . 0.05 gm
$Al_2(SO_4)_3$ . . . . 0.05 gm

$CuSO_4 \bullet 5H_2O$	0.05 gm
$NiSO_4 \bullet 6H_2O$	0.05 gm
$Co(NO_3)_2 \bullet 6H_2O$	0.05 gm
KI	0.03 gm
LiCl	0.03 gm
KBr	0.03 gm
TiO_2	0.03 gm
$SnCl_2 \bullet 2H_2O$	0.03 gm

The experimental group solutions should be prepared from the formula of the control solution, omitting one mineral. Containers should be carefully labeled, and seedlings should be observed periodically so that the effects of mineral deficiency, if any, can be observed.

The interconnection of water and minerals can be stressed in a discussion of the solvent properties of water and in the permeability of membranes.

Many experiments can be performed to examine the importance of sunlight on plants. The process of photosynthesis can again be connected to oxygen production. The discussion of water can also include the fact that soils vary in consistency and may not retain water or may hold it too firmly, such as the absorption of water by clay. Obviously all of these factors play a part in the survial of plants.

2. *What About Man?* Here the many problems of increased populations can be explored for their relationship to plant conservation. The very expansion of communities and the resultant clearing of lands has destroyed the natural habitat of many plant species.

Soil pollution from the dumping of wastes has killed many plants and will prevent their growth for years to come. Air pollution causes the destruction of flowers and even whole plants. Hydrofluoric acid, sulfur dioxide, ozone, and ethylene all can kill plants. The flowers on a healthy plant have been known to die completely in the ten-minute trip through the Holland Tunnel connecting New York City and New Jersey. Polluted water passing through soil can kill plants and alter soil chemistry for the future. Man, through the overuse of resources, poor planning and indiscriminate flower picking, adds to this destruction.

To investigate soil and water pollution, students can plan controlled experiments with potted plants such as the geranium. Mixing a "pollutant" of their choice with the soil of one plant, or watering a plant with laboratory-prepared or field-gathered polluted water will provide data on subsequent plant growth or changes. (Students should make certain to use a second plant as a control.) Information on the effects of air pollution on plants can be gathered by contacting botanical gardens located in areas of heavy pollution. The Brooklyn Botanic Garden, for example, identifies those plants which are suited for survival in polluted air in its 1971 publication on shrubs and trees.

3. *What About Endangered Species?*   Students should be asked to assemble a display of sketches and literature on rare plants of their state. This information can be obtained from state conservation groups and government agencies. The county agricultural agent or nearby college or university could probably provide the specific sources of their area. It is important to remind students that there are protected plant species which cannot be removed from the sites on which they are growing without special permission. This fact will stress the dependence of some plants on particular types of soil, nutrients, microbes, or other environmental conditions. This will also illustrate the problems faced by plants which have not adapted to a changing environment. Examples of common plants can be used to show that adaptability enables some species to exist under a wide range of conditions, while other plants need extremely specific conditions for survival. Some orchids can live in soil only when certain microbes are present.

The class can consider the ways in which plant species are lost, including the increased clearing of land for houses, the needless picking or uprooting of plants by thoughtless people, and disruptions in the balance of nature as members in the food chain are eliminated or added. If such a program exists, they might gather information about the conditions under which private citizens can collect and raise wild flowers and other endangered species. It would not be advisable for students to attempt this themselves unless they have expert supervision. Students must be made fully aware of not doing damage in the name of a "laboratory exercise."

As a final project, students can be requested to prepare reports on rare and/or endangered plants, using sources such as *National Geographic* magazine and the many botanical and horticultural magazines available. These can be obtained and used at the library of any local botanical garden. The lesson can be concluded with a discussion of the interrelationship of plants and animals. *Since we cannot manufacture our own food what happens to a wildlife community when plants die?*

What Can You Do?

1. Have your parents press for and support legislative measures that will preserve natural park lands and habitats. There are very few of these natural habitats left in our rapidly growing environment.
2. Do not needlessly pick or uproot plants. This can disrupt the balance of nature, as well as cause the loss of rare or endangered species.

Pertinent Facts

1. Water, minerals, and sunlight are all important to the growth and development of plants.
2. Many of the aspects of ecology such as water, air, and soil pollution affect the survival of plants.
3. Man helps to destroy plants not only by his pollution but also by clearing land, by altering the balance of nature, and by careless picking and destruction of individual plants.

Possible Quiz

1. What are the essential materials needed for plant survival? In what process are they crucial?
2. Identify three forms of pollution and indicate how they affect plant conservation.
3. Describe a controlled experiment you would perform to study the effects of pollution on plants.

4. In what ways can endangered species be protected and saved from extinction?
5. Discuss any one of the class reports on rare or endangered plants giving some information about its habitat and life cycle.

READINGS

DeBach, Paul (ed.), *Biological Control of Insect Pests and Weeds.* New York: Rheinhold Publishing Co., 1964.

Edwards, Clive A., "Soil Pollutants and Soil Animals." *Scientific American,* Vol. 220, No. 4, April, 1969.

Elton, Charles S., *The Ecology of Invasions by Animals and Plants.* New York: John Wiley and Sons, 1958.

Smith, Robert L., *Ecology and Field Biology.* New York: Harper and Row, Inc., 1966.

FILMS

"Conservation and Our Forests." 15 minutes, sound, color, $5.75. University of Michigan, A-V Education Center, 416 Fourth Street, Ann Arbor, Michigan 48103.

"Man Makes a Desert." 11 minutes, sound, color $9.25. University of Michigan.

LESSON 10

Animal Conservation

Lesson time: 45 minutes

Aim

To describe how man can protect endangered animal life from extinction using knowledge of the man-made threats to animal species.

Materials

films and slides

Planned Lesson

1. *What Factors Threaten Animal Survival?*   Students should understand that wildlife is important not as game for sportsmen but as an important indicator of the quality of the environment in which man lives. They may already be familar with the effects of DDT on the calcium deposits in bird eggs. This chemical alters the bird metabolism so that calcium is not adequately deposited in the shell and the eggs are destroyed as the parent birds sit on them in the hatching process. Interested students might report on the likely extinction of some species as a result of the effect of this pesticide.

Water pollution has greatly affected fish and other aquatic organisms. The classic "dead Lake Erie" has been written about many times and might be an interesting topic of discussion. The

85

oil pollution of water has also been well documented in articles dealing with the Santa Barbara oil slicks. In each case the *Reader's Guide to Periodic Literature* should provide a multitude of sources for interested students.

The State Fish and Game Department or its equivalent in your town can be called upon for local information and will often provide a guest speaker and slides which illustrate damage to wildlife and preventative techniques.

2. *What Is the Chief Cause of Reduced Wildlife Populations?* Many suggestions will be offered, but students will be surprised to note that loss of habitat is the major problem. Again, this can be connected with the whole problem of increased human population and the need for more living space, more airports, more roads, more garbage dumps and more of everything. The obvious result is less unspoiled land for breeding and feeding. *The National Wildlife Magazine* (August-September, 1969) suggests that most endangered species are in trouble because of diminishing habitats. Each state has its own specific problems in this area which can be studied with the help of local and state agencies including the Fish and Game Department.

Special emphasis might be placed on waste disposal problems (see lesson 16) as it is involved here. As cities run out of space for dumping waste, they frequently consider filling in shallow bodies of water thus destroying marsh lands which are essential for survival for many forms of life. New York City's plan to fill Jamaica Bay and the resultant opposition is a case in point.

A tragic but very important aspect of animal conservation has to do with the plight of the spotted cat. Because of man's desire to use their skins for coats, wall hangings, and rugs, many spotted cats are near extinction, and some experts feel that some may be beyond help. Students need to consider the arguments sometimes given in defense of those who buy and wear such clothing. They say that the coat was already made, the five or more cats needed to supply the pelts were killed long ago, and therefore the buyer is not guilty of their deaths. Perhaps not, but the buyer is directly responsible for the order by the store owner to replace the coat that was sold. This order assures the death of the tigers, leopards, or other cats which will be used to make the new coat. It should be noted that many fur dealers have voluntarily stopped trading in furs of endangered species. A survey of local fur shops may prove to be a very valuable learning experience.

The seal problem is another case. A great deal of publicity has been given to the clubbing of baby seals in Canada and the skinning of the babies which may still be alive, while the mothers look on. Photographs have been printed in magazines showing large areas of lands covered with the bodies of skinned seals. Students may have seen advertisements which explain that a particular tribe of Alaskan Indians have exclusive treaty rights with the United States government to hunt adult seals and that they are taken by humane methods. The advertisements go on to point out that this is the main source of income of the tribe and is also an important control on the size of seal herds. This type of article juxtaposed with the ones on seal clubbings can serve as the basis of good class discussions.

3. *What About the Future?* Here one good source of current and projected information is the National Wildlife "Environmental Quality Index." The Department of Interior and its main branches such as the National Parks Service can also provide specific information.

The teacher should point out that some species are irreversibly headed for extinction because their current population, even fully protected, cannot produce enough new organisms to keep pace with natural deaths. Some whales and spotted cats might already be in that category. Other organisms are probably moving toward extinction because of irreversible damage by pollution as in the case of some birds. Others have responded well to efforts to save them. A particularly interesting story is that of the trumpeter swans fed regularly at a desolate Canadian lake by three generations of one family. The swans have made a spectacular recovery. Many accounts of this study have appeared in recent years and can be located in local sources by checking the *Reader's Guide to Periodic Literature.*

Students might consult sources to learn about species which are doing well, such as small game, white-tailed deer, and American buffalo (bison). Here again is the interesting story of a species nearly gone which was saved by careful management. The bison herds are now large enough to maintain herd size.

As a concluding activity the teacher can relate all of the

facets of increased population to the animal conservation problem. Each lesson can be used to add to and further develop the closely intertwined and interdependent aspects of the ecological crisis.

What Can You Do?

1. Tell your parents and friends not to buy or wear garments made from the fur or skins of wild animals.
2. Do not wear such things as alligator shoes or belts. Purchase and wear only the hides of those animals that are specifically raised for their fur or that have been specifically slaughtered for their meat.
3. Together with family, friends, and neighbors, support the endangered species of animals. Form citizens groups in defense of these endangered species.
4. Do not hunt these animals, and above all, do not destroy their homes and natural habitats.

Pertinent Facts

1. The success of wildlife is a direct indication of man's environment.
2. The most serious threat to wildlife is the loss of habitat.
3. Man's ego need to have rare and exotic possessions has helped to make some species extinct and is moving others in that direction.

Possible Quiz

1. What environmental factors contribute to the extinction of an animal species?
2. Discuss the effect of the loss of habitat on a species.
3. Identify some ways in which you could contribute to the effort to save endangered species.
4. Describe or discuss some ways in which various organizations are helping to overcome wildlife extinction.

5. Discuss two ways by which individuals contribute to the extinction of animal species.

READINGS

"Index of Environmental Quality." *National Wildlife Magazine.* August-September 1970. Washington, D.C. National Wildlife Federation.

U.S. Department of the Interior, Fish and Wildlife Service, Washington, D.C. (Ask for current publications).

U.S. Department of the Interior, National Park Service, Washington, D.C. (Ask for current publications).

FILMS

"Conserving Our Wildlife Today." 11 minutes, sound, color, $4.00. University of Michigan, A-V Education Center, 416 Fourth Street, Ann Arbor, Michigan 48103.

"Our Endangered Wildlife." 51 minutes, sound, color, $35.00. McGraw-Hill Text Films, 330 W. 42nd Street, New York, 10036.

"Poisons, Pests, and People." 44 minutes, black and white, sound, $16.00. McGraw-Hill Contemporary Film Rental Office, 330 W. 42nd Street, New York, New York, 10036.

LESSON 11

Water Conservation

Lesson time: 45 minutes

Aim

To estimate water consumption on a national or world-wide basis from measurements of water consumption in personal daily life and to develop solutions for the conservation of our diminishing water supply.

Materials

films
crayon marking pencil

Planned Lesson

1. *How Does Water Get from the Ocean to the Land?* The lesson can begin with a general discussion of the uses of water and a consideration of the hydrologic cycle. This cycle could be summarized by beginning with the principal reservoir of water, the oceans. It must be pointed out that although the ocean is salt water, evaporation involves only the water, not the salts. As a result, this water ultimately condenses as fresh water. Rainfall, then, is not salt water.

Some specific discussion of the great amounts of water used in food production should be included. Many plants use large quantities of water, amounts which may be measured in hundreds of quarts or gallons per growing season. The interrelation between animals and the plants they eat should be explored. The water use of the plant plus that of the animal eating the plant can be tallied. A number of references provide information about the number of quarts of water per growing season needed by various crops. For example, a pound of wheat uses about sixty gallons of water, a pound of meat requires 2,500-6,000 gallons. From this the class can conclude that agriculture demands large amounts of water; the countries with the most serious food problems in attempting to increase food production constantly put a strain on their water supply.

Student reports could be developed on the various uses of water, including the amounts involved. They should research the many industrial processes which use large amounts of water, prepare lists of industries, and indicate how the water is used.

Class discussion should consider that more than ninety-five percent of the earth's water supply is salt water and that most of the fresh water is frozen in the polar ice caps. *What would happen if the polar ice caps melted? Would this be a way to increase our fresh water supply?* This can lead to study of the ground water supply which is currently being tapped extensively for irrigation purposes. Other important points to be considered would be projects for irrigation of arid lands and the possibility of desalting of water. In each case it would be important to consider the economic factors involved. Obviously irrigation water for arid areas would need to be transported, making it expensive. Desalting, of course, involves the building of plants which cost money.

These and related subjects, such as projects which attempt to link water use with more efficient food production, might be considered in greater detail if the teacher wishes.

It will be important to stress the effects of increased population on water conservation. Lesson 1 can be tied in effectively. The problems of sewage plants dumping effluents into streams, increased industrial waste entering bodies of water, oil spills, and all the many other industrial problems should be brought into the picture.

2. *How Can We Help to Conserve Water?*   This question should be fully explored in all its ramifications. First, a list can be

developed from class discussion which suggests the ways in which the class members use water. The nature of the list will vary from area to area but generally it will include recreational uses, agricultural and/or gardening uses, cooking, cleaning, and related uses. Each can then be considered separately with student and teacher suggestions for ways in which water can be conserved. Some of these might include measuring the amount of water used when taking a bath as compared with a shower. The individual can use a *crayon* marking pencil, a child's crayon, or even a thick soap mark to measure the line of bath water. (Students should remember that some materials may stain the tub.) *Should you measure this level while you are in the tub? Why not?* A moment might be devoted to Archimedes' principle. This should not take long since students will have observed that the water level rises when objects are placed in a water-filled container. It will be necessary only to briefly review the concept of displacement. *How can you compare this with the amount of water used when you take a shower? Is it more economical to take a bath or a shower?* It would be interesting to tabulate results as gathered by students perhaps using inches of water as a method of tabulation. Other specific suggestions could be to check faucets for leaks. The class can study this loss by adjusting a faucet to drip water and to then collect it during a timed interval. *How much water is lost in an hour? If 100 homes in your community had such a leak which was not repaired for one week, how much water would be lost?*

Using the suggestion that a brick be carefully placed in the reservoir tank of each toilet, the teacher can bring in Archimedes' principle again. *Why does this save water? Why does it not reduce the operation of the toilet?* Discussion can range widely on this topic. Other aspects for consideration are: letting water run until cold, watering a garden as opposed to using plants which can do well on local rainfall levels, and checking all pipes and connections for leaks.

Student reports or guest speakers might be used to review local, state, and federal water conservation plans. While somewhat dated, the Department of Agriculture Handbook, "Water" (1955), will be a very useful reference. An individual or group should be encouraged to contact the United Nations for material on irrigation projects and other water-related work. Some might contact the Department of Agriculture for information on federal programs and perhaps even foreign governments which have attempted to work on water conservation. Perhaps a discussion of a project such as the Aswan Dam can be included. This can be expanded to consider the related disease problems, changes in land fertility, and other aspects which are not strictly part of water conservation studies.

In conclusion, the group can consider the many commercial aspects of water conservation, such as the use of large rubber sheets to create artificial lakes. Many advertisements run in magazines, for example, can be found relating to this. Letters to oil and chemical companies can be used by students to research this topic further.

What Can You Do?

1. Take brief showers instead of taking a bath. It is more economical. You can save as much as fifteen to twenty gallons of water this way.
2. Make certain that your faucets do not leak. You can lose as many as twenty to thirty gallons of water a day this way.
3. Check all pipes and connections in your home for leaks.
4. Do not wash dishes in running water.
5. Do not let water run until it becomes cold. If you want cold water for drinking purposes keep a bottle of water in your refrigerator.
6. Carefully place a brick in the reservoir tank of your toilet. This will cut down in the amount of water wasted with each flush, but will not impair the efficiency of the flush.
7. When you plan your garden, use plants that will do well on local rainfall levels. This will cut down on the need for watering your garden often.

Pertinent Facts

1. Water is a reusable resource which is constantly moving through the hydrologic cycle.
2. Thousands of gallons of water are needed to produce a pound of meat. This represents the water which produced the vegetation the animal ate as well as the water the animal itself used.
3. Only a tiny fraction of the earth's water is available for our immediate use.
4. Water conservation involves a great many aspects including control of industrial uses and complete treatment of sewage.
5. Water conservation is extremely important because we are using our chief source, the ground water, at a very rapid rate.

Possible Quiz

1. Briefly explain the hydrologic cycle. How does salt water become fresh?
2. Why is the need for water so crucial in countries such as India?
3. Why is it not feasible to consider melting the polar ice caps for water?
4. What are some factors which work against the conservation of water?
5. What can we as individuals do to help in water conservation?

READINGS

Addison, Herbert, *Land, Water and Food.* London: Chapman and Hall, 1961.

Clawson, M., H.H. Landsberg, and L.T. Alexander, "Desalted Seawater for Agriculture: Is It Economic?" *Science.* Vol. 164, 1969.

U.S. Department of Agriculture, "Water." Washington, D.C., 1955.

FILMS

"Element Three." 46 minutes, color, sound, $25.00. International Film Bureau, 332 South Michigan Avenue, Chicago, Illinois 60604.

"Problems of Conservation: Water." 16 minutes, sound, color, $8.00. Encyclopedia Britannica Films, Inc., 1150 Wilmette Avenue, Wilmette, Illinois 60091.

Biological Controls and Their Relationship to the Environment

UNIT 3

LESSON 12

The Biological
Effects of Pesticides

Lesson time: 45 minutes

Aim

To determine the harmful and beneficial effects of pesticides on the environment and the organism from readings, and to postulate the alternatives if mankind is to survive.

Materials

films

Planned Lesson

1. *What Are the Effects of Pesticides?* The purpose of this lesson should be to specifically consider the effects of pesticides rather than their nature or uses. The material in Lesson 5 should be reviewed as preparation. It can then be assumed by the teacher that the students are aware of the various categories of pesticides and the uses of each.

Students should be asked to develop a list of plant and animal diseases caused by pests, primarily by insects. *Why can we limit ourselves to insects?* It should be emphasized that pesticides are used, for the most part, against insects and rodents and that plant and animal diseases caused by pests are usually traceable to insects. The lists should also include carrier and causative agents. For example, African sleeping sickness is caused by a protozoan carried by certain mosquitoes. The list could be quite long, including Dutch elm disease, malaria, tapeworm infestation, cucumber wilt, yellow fever, Rocky Mountain spotted fever, typhus and bubonic plague. This activity should be a rather dramatic display of the importance of pesticides in the controlling of disease. To further emphasize the point, the teacher might present the example of Ceylon. Until 1945, a great many deaths in Ceylon were due to malaria. The death rate from malaria was twenty-two per thousand in 1945. In 1946, DDT was introduced to control the disease-carrying mosquitoes. In 1969, the continuing reduction in the death rate had reached the low point of eight per thousand. Since then concern over the ecological pollution associated with DDT has led to a sharp curtailment of the program. The World Health Organization soon reported a sharp increase in the number of malaria deaths.

2. *Can We Do Without Pesticides?* It is very important for the teacher to help students to develop a mature attitude which will allow them to consider both sides of the question intelligently and unemotionally. They must realize that there is a need for pesticides but that they must be carefully controlled.

A great deal of publicity has been given to the dangers of using pesticides. These should be thoroughly investigated so that students can move toward a truly scientific attitude of thought. Both *Silent Spring* and *Since Silent Spring* should be required preparatory reading. DDT might be selected as an example with emphasis on its long and widespread use. Many resources provide statistics on parts per million (ppm) of DDT detected in species far removed from areas of DDT use, difficulties with calcium metabolism in birds resulting in egg breakage before hatching (and subsequent danger of extinction in many cases), dangers to salmon, trout and other fish, and the serious imbalances created in ecosystems. Some researchers believe, for example, that mites have become a serious problem only because their natural predators have been greatly reduced in numbers by pesticides. The mites therefore can multiply without control by their predators. From their readings, students will learn that a large number of animals including mammals can and have been killed by insecticides. It should be noted that some research has been done (Wurster) which suggests that DDT may also reduce the rate of photosynthesis in phytoplankton. Since these minute plants are the basis of the food chains in the water, the implications are clear. Review of this material can most easily be done by having students consider the ways in which organisms pick up pesticides through soil, water, and other organisms. They should also gather information about length of time needed for major pesticides to be broken down to harmless end products.

3. *What Alternatives Are There?*   The concept of biological control can be introduced as a logical possibility. If students have done outside reading concerning pesticide dangers, they have no doubt come across some strong criticisms of pesticides on the grounds that they destroy nontarget organisms and otherwise upset the ecological balance. *How can scientists take advantage of biological considerations to control an insect?* Students might suggest using chemicals to alter its life cycle. These might be used to sterilize large numbers of males and then releasing them so that the females they mate with will lay unfertilized eggs. Perhaps scientists might synthesize sex attractants which normally lure males to females for mating. The synthesized attractants could be used to capture large numbers of males and thereby prevent many matings. Chemical sterilants might be introduced into the food supply. These and many other possibilities are, for the most part, still experimental. The use of natural enemies is not. There are many cases where this has been successful. It is important to point out that this should be done only after careful study to prevent the introduction of an organism which itself might become a pest or which will seriously damage the ecological balance. A third encouraging area of study is the use of microbes as natural controls. A great deal of work has been done in this area and some microbial controls have been used successfully for years. This would provide a fascinating area of library research for interested students.

The teacher should help students to realize that not all pesticides are equally toxic nor do they function in the same manner. They should be used with great caution and with understanding of the impact they have on ecology; and, other methods of pest control should be used whenever possible.

What Can You Do?

1. Warn your parents and friends about the dangers of pesticides. Have them cut down on the pesticides they are now using.
2. Have your parents explore the possibility of using biological controls in place of pesticides.
3. Do not use chlorinated hydrocarbons. They are the most dangerous of the pesticides.

Pertinent Facts

1. Botanical compounds such as rotenone and pyrethrum break down quickly in the soil while chlorinated hydrocarbons like DDT persist for years.
2. Insects can do a great deal of damage both by destroying vegetation and by carrying disease.
3. Many scientists feel that biological control procedures have not yet developed to the point where we can do away with all insecticide use, but they agree that they should be used with great care.
4. Biological controls include use of knowledge about life cycles; to sterilize, lure, or otherwise prevent males from mating with females successfully; use of natural predators; and use of microbial agents.

Possible Quiz

1. Identify five diseases carried by insects, the insect itself, and the actual causative agent.
2. Give some examples of the harmful effects of pesticides.
3. Beginning with the phytoplankton, trace a possible path for a molecule of DDT as it passes through the food chain.

4. What are the advantages and disadvantages of introducing natural enemies to control pests?
5. What methods are being developed for future insect
control?

READINGS

de Bach, Paul, *Biological Control of Insects, Pests, and Weeds.* New York:
Rheinhold, 1965.

Carson, Rachel, *Silent Spring,* Boston: Houghton-Mifflin, 1962.

Edwards, Clive A., "Soil Pollutants and Soil Animals," *Scientific American.*
Vol. 220, No. 4, April, 1969.

Knipling, E.F., "The Eradication of the Screw-Worm Fly," *Scientific American.* Vol. 203, No. 54, 1960.

Wurster, Charles F. Jr., "DDT Reduces Photosynthesis by Marine Phytoplankton," *Science.* Vol. 158, 1968.

FILMS

"DDT—Knowing It Survives Us." 30 minutes, sound, color, fee not known.
Time-Life Films, Room 33-36 Time-Life Building, Rockefeller Center,
New York, N.Y. 10020.

"The Kitfox—Vanishing Species." Sound, color, $12.00 Journal Films, 909
West Diversey Parkway, Chicago, Illinois 60614.

"By Land, Sea, and Air." Sound, color, $5.00 per day. Citizenship Council,
Legislative Department, Oil, Chemical, and Atomic Workers International Union, 1126 16th Street N.W., Washington, D.C. 20036.

"Poisons, Pests, and People." 55 minutes, sound, black and white, $16.00.
McGraw-Hill Contemporary Film Rental Office, 330 West 42nd Street,
New York, N.Y. 10018.

LESSON 13

Radiation and You

Lesson time: 45 minutes
Laboratory time: 90 minutes

AIM

To investigate the benefits and harmful effects of radiation on the environment, on the cell, and on man.

MATERIALS

films

PLANNED LESSON

1. *What Is Radioactivity?* A review of Lesson 7 would be extremely helpful to this study. The teacher will need to review the nature of the three forms of radioactivity, alpha, beta, and gamma rays, and should also reintroduce the units of measurement: roentgen and rem. Students should know that a roentgen is a measure of numbers of ions produced per cubic centimeter of air and that a rem (roentgen equivalent in man) represents a dose of any type radiation which produces a biological effect equivalent to the absorption of one roentgen of radiation.

Beginning with the benefits of radiation, food preservation

105

would be an important use for irradiation which has a direct effect on the individual. *What use can be made of the fact that specific doses of radiation can inhibit sprouting, kill insects, and kill bacteria without damaging the foods so treated?* It might be mentioned that it was once believed that irradiated foods were poisonous, but this has since been proven incorrect. Irradiated meats can be kept for many months at room temperature. Students could be asked to develop a list of other foods which have been preserved by this method. *What other purposes might this serve? Could irradiation be used in Customs control of foods?*

2. *How Is It Used?*   The laboratory activities of Lesson 7 will be well suited to use here as introduction to some of the agricultural uses of irradiation. The study of the movement of water in a plant, for example, can be done in class. "Tagging" of molecules with radioactive materials and their use in studying plant metabolism can be considered. The use of radioactive tags on insects to follow their movements can also be covered. The World Health Organization can provide information on various programs using such methods. They will also have material on the use of irradiation to induce earlier germination in seeds.

The commercial uses of radiation can be studied by having committees contact local or national companies to ask if they use radioactive sensors and for what purpose. They will be surprised at the wide range of such uses. They could obtain the name of a manufacturer of such equipment and contact them for materials. A number of companies provide a wide range of materials including free films.

The discussion can be concluded with a look at the more familiar medical and dental uses of radiation including X-ray pictures, X-ray therapy to destroy unwanted cells, and the use of radioisotopes to study the metabolism of the various tissues of the body.

3. *What About Dangers?*   Exposure to radiation must be carefully measured to prevent overdoses. Monitoring equipment can be provided by local Civil Defense units. These might include film badges, dosimeters, and the variety of elaborate machines which can monitor an entire body. *What is an acceptable level of exposure?* Recalling that roentgen and rem are both based on the production of ions/unit volume of air, students should be able to

suggest that the presence of these ions will inevitably alter the chemistry of the cells in which the ions are produced. It should be obvious that a single large dose would be more dangerous than a series of smaller doses over a period of time. A lethal dose of radiation is indicated as LD_{50-30}. That is, the amount of radiation that would kill 50 percent of a population within 30 days. Estimates of a human lethal dose vary from 400 to 700 roentgens and perhaps even higher. *Why is it not known what the level is?* The inability to test this should be brought in although it should also be mentioned that X-ray therapy has provided some information about radiation tolerance.

4. *How Does Radiation Affect the Cell and Organism?* Using their knowledge of cell physiology, students should suggest possible results of exposure to radiation on the cell. The teacher can help to develop a list including possible destruction of enzymes, chromosome breakage, swelling of the nucleus, swelling of the entire cell, increased viscosity of protoplasm, and increased membrane permeability, clogging of capillaries with broken cells, and delayed or blocked mitosis. Students are usually interested in the actual results of overexposure. This would provide an interesting report project or the teacher might prefer to simply list the characteristics. They would include (for chronic local exposure) reddening of skin, blistering, formation of very slow-healing lesions, loss of hair, possible cancerous growths, genetic effects, and a decrease in leukocytes. (If a massive dose of radiation is received, the number of white blood cells goes up rather than down.) *Why is this?* Although individual response varies, there are generally four phases of "radiation sickness":

1. Nausea, vomiting, general lassitude.
2. A few days or weeks of general well-being (this is shorter with larger doses).
3. Reaction peaks—prostration, loss of appetite, loss of weight, fever, rapid heart action, severe diarrhea, bleeding of the gums, loss of hair (this may last for days or weeks). Survival depends on ability to withstand this phase.
4. If phase three is survived, there is a long recovery

period, blood may be altered for a long time, the individual may ultimately develop leukemia and/or cataracts.

The blood changes which accompany radiation exposure occur because the bone marrow and the lymph are particularly sensitive to radiation. Generally there is an initial increase in leukocyte level followed by a sharp drop. Since the white blood cells fight infection, this means that the individual is more susceptible to infections. The number of platelets also drops which interferes with clotting. *Why is bone tissue said to be radio-sensitive?* The teacher might mention that reproductive organs and the gastrointestinal tract are also very sensitive to radiation while muscle, nerve tissue, and fully grown bone is radioresistant. Skin, kidneys, liver, and lungs are intermediate.

Although not as common as external exposure to radiation, the class should also consider the implications of internal exposure by inhaling or ingesting radioactive materials.

5.*Genetic Effects.*   Using a review of DNA structure as a foundation, class discussion should develop the idea that ionizing radiation causes random changes in DNA structure. The teacher might use a complex machine, such as a car or television set, to show that a random change in any complex system, whether biological or mechanical, is more likely to be harmful than beneficial. *What defects might occur?* Since the damage is random, students can develop the idea that any defect is possible, but that many probably will be so serious that if an egg or sperm is so damaged, it may never develop if involved in the production of a zygote.

A review should include a general overview of the importance of radiation to the individual. Student committees can arrange visits to medical facilities to see X-ray equipment and therapy equipment and to hear lectures on the use of equipment and treatment for radiation sickness.

What Can You Do?

1. Do not knowingly expose yourself to radioactive substances or to sources of radiation.

2. When you go for dental X-rays make certain that a lead apron or other similar protective device covers that part of your body that is not being X-rayed.
3. Do not sit too closely to appliances (such as television sets or radar ovens) which may emit radiation. Have these appliances checked periodically to insure that they are not emitting dangerously high levels of radioactivity.

Pertinent Facts

1. Radiation can be used to preserve food.
2. Plant and animal metabolism can be studied by using radioisotopes.
3. Radiation can cause damage to chromosomes, swelling of cells, changes in membrane permeability and increased protoplasm viscosity.
4. Human beings respond to overdoses of radiation by developing a series of symptoms including nausea, diarrhea, loss of hair, and sometimes death.
5. The less evident but equally serious effects of radiation exposure include changes in blood composition, possible development of leukemia, and development of cataracts.

Possible Quiz

1. List four ways in which radioactivity can be used to help us.
2. Why would irradiation of all luggage passing through Customs be of value?
3. Why is it that the level of a lethal dose of radiation for human beings is not known?
4. What are some of the effects of radiation on cells? On the organism?
5. Why are some tissues said to be radiosensitive? Which ones are radiosensitive? Which are radioresistant?

READINGS

Curtis, Richard and Elizabeth Hogan, *Perils of the Peaceful Atom: The Myth of Safe Nuclear Power Plants.* New York: Doubleday, 1969.

Glasstone, Samuel, *Sourcebook in Atomic Energy,* second edition. New York: Van Nostrand, 1968.

Harrison, G.A., J.S. Weiner, J.M. Tanner and N.A. Barnicot, *Human Biology.* New York: Oxford University Press, 1964.

Lerner, I. Michael, *Heredity, Evolution, and Society.* San Francisco: Freeman, 1968.

Novick, Sheldon, *The Careless Atom.* Boston: Houghton-Mifflin, 1969.

FILMS

"Enter with Caution: The Atomic Age." Two parts, 26 minutes each, sound, black and white, $17.00. Association Films, 600 Madison Avenue, New York, N.Y. 10022.

"The Fallout Atom." 26 minutes, (no price). Association Films.

"Nuclear Radiation Fallout." 15 minutes, color, sound, $5.65. Anco Educational Films.

LESSON 14

Food Consumption:
Diminishing Returns

Lesson time: 45 minutes

Aim

To be able to construct laboratory ecological communities based on the concepts of food chains and food pyramids, and to generalize the effects of an ever-increasing population on food supply.

Materials

    films
    terrarium

Planned Lesson

1. *Food Chains.* The concept of food chains beginning with the essential green plants should be reviewed. It would also be helpful to review the process of photosynthesis in order to point out that this process can use carbon dioxide and water as the raw materials for the production of glucose.

111

Stated simply, photosynthesis can be said to be the food-making process of plants in which sugar and oxygen are produced from water, carbon dioxide, and energy in the form of light, in the presence of chlorophyll.

Reference should be made to the role of chlorophyll in photosynthesis. Briefly, students should be familiarized with the functioning of a catalyst. Chlorophyll may be used as a specific example. It is unnecessary to go into great detail here. The points which should be mentioned include that a biological catalyst, or enzyme, is a chemical which speeds up, or makes possible, some chemical change; that the enzyme is not used up during the change and remains chemically the same afterward, so that it can be reused a number of times before "wearing out"; and that each enzyme has a single specific function within a chemical reaction (the Lock and Key Theory).

Students should be aware that, in addition to the green chlorophyll, many plants also contain carotene, a deep orange pigment, and xanthophyll, a bright yellow pigment. These, together with other accessory plant pigments, play a role in leaf coloration. Little is known concerning the specific functions of these pigments.

The teacher should also bring out the fact that there are two main phases in the process of photosynthesis—the light reaction and the dark reaction. The light reaction (Hill reaction) is a light-driven reaction which consists of the photochemical decomposition of water. This decomposition of water by light is also known as photolysis.

The dark reaction is so named, not because it must take place in the dark, but rather because it can occur in the dark. That is, light is not essential. The dark reaction involves the fixation of carbon dioxide to produce organic compounds such as sugar. The hydrogen produced by photolysis combines with the carbon and oxygen of carbon dioxide. The relationship of the two stages should now be evident.

The film, "The Sea," is a very good one to use in conjunction with this lesson. It traces the food chains from the phytoplankton and zooplankton to larger and larger species, as one feeds on the other. The film then shows that death and decay by bacteria ultimately converts the organism into the raw materials which can be used by the phytoplankton. The chain can be identified as producers (green plants), primary consumers (herbivores), secondary consumers (carnivores), tertiary consumers (carnivores which eat carnivores) and so. These can be said to make up levels, the first level being the producers, the second those animals which eat producers (herbivores), and the third level those animals which eat herbivores (carnivores).

2. *What About Energy Stored in Food Chains?* Calling upon their knowledge of cellular respiration, students should recall that the Kreb's Cycle is not 100 percent efficient, and that some energy is lost as molecules are broken down.

Photosynthesis, of course, traps and stores energy from light. As each step of the food chain occurs, energy is lost, which explains the figures quoted in Lesson 11. These figures state, for example, that thousands of pounds of grain may be used to produce one tenth as much (a thousand pounds) of beef, which in turn may produce only one lightweight human being.

The class should be helped to understand that by changing levels in the food chain, we can greatly decrease or increase the amount of food required to develop certain organisms. Thus, it can be seen that as one moves to higher levels, there are, indeed, diminishing returns.

A classroom terrarium or aquarium might be set up by a student or group of students, showing several levels of a food chain. Some very helpful hints in developing such a terrarium are listed below.

Suitable containers include battery jars, wide-mouth gallon jars, old aquaria, or specially purchased terraria cases. A large rectangular case would be the simplest to use. It should have a cover of glass to prevent excessive evaporation. Care should be taken not to seal this cover, in order that air may circulate freely.

Many ecological principles can be observed and studied by the development of several different kinds of terraria. Students should be encouraged to determine what factors must be controlled to maintain proper environmental conditions. Conditions will vary, depending upon the types of specimens to be kept. In general, there are four main types of terraria, classified in terms of climate conditions. These include swamp, bog, woodland, and desert habitats. The conditions required for each of the main types are as follows.

A. *Swampy.* A shallow pool of water should be created in the terrarium. The soil on the side of the terrarium should be several inches above the water line. If possible, soil from a swampy area should be transported to the classroom and placed in the terrarium on top of a base layer of gravel. A layer of living or dead sphagnum should be placed over this as a top layer. Pieces of charcoal should be added to the gravel. The layer of gravel provides drainage, while the garden soil-sphagnum mixture provides an acid soil. The bits of charcoal absorb odors. After the soil is placed in the terrarium it should be thoroughly soaked.

The swampy terrarium is an excellent place in which to raise insectivorous plants. The care of these plants depends upon the species. Although all insectivorous plants require a moist or aquatic environment, there are differences. Sundews generally grow on moss-covered rocks or logs above the surface of the water, rarely in contact with it; the Venus-flytrap requires a moist soil with good drainage; the pitcher plant must have at least a few of its roots in water. All require an acid soil, usually growing in sphagnum or peat moss bogs.

To protect these plants from the dry air of the heated classroom, the humidity in the terrarium should be kept high. Although some sunlight is necessary, excessive amounts will cause damage and may even kill the plants. They must be observed frequently when the terrarium is first established, to determine proper sunlight requirements. It will take approximately two weeks after planting for new plant growth to become apparent.

The pool of water in the terrarium might contain insect larvae and small fish or tadpoles. If large enough, this pool can be set up, like any small aquarium, with plants and fish.

B. *Bog.* The preparation of base and soil in a bog terrarium is the same as in a swampy terrarium. The chief difference in physical condition is the amount of water. Here excess water should be restricted to the gravel layer which should always contain some water. Bog plants of various types, as well as insectivorous plants, will do well here. Animals which would be suitable include all small amphibians (newts, toads, salamanders).

C. *Woodland.* The most versatile terrarium is the woodland arrangement. A great number of plants and animals do well here. The preparation should include a base of gravel, sand, and humus well mixed. Regular potting soil should then be placed on this base. The size and number of animal specimens will depend upon the size of the terrarium. Care must be used in the selection and arrangement of plant specimens. Most small animals of the woodland will do well in this terrarium. They include beetles, snails, snakes, frogs, lizards, and toads.

D. *Desert.* This is the simplest of all types to prepare and maintain. The base should be composed of about two inches of coarse sand. This should then be covered with fine desert sand, which can be purchased from most pet shops or commercial supply houses. The base layer should be moistened, but the top layer should be kept dry. A small pan for water should be embedded in the sand so that it is level with the sand surface. Cactus plants should now be planted in a pleasing arrangement. The area around the plants should be lightly watered when planting is complete. A few attractive rocks and a piece of driftwood might be included if there is adequate space. Some snakes do well in a desert terrarium, as do certain lizards. Other desert creatures might be used instead. Since humidity should not be high, no cover of glass is needed. A piece of wire mesh over the top will be enough to keep in the animals. Make certain that the mesh is secured so that it cannot be pushed aside by the animals.

Students must pay special attention to the interrelationships among all the specimens when planning the terraria. As proper soil, water, and temperature will generally insure satisfactory plant growth, this is perhaps a simpler problem than that of the animals in the terraria. Students should be aware of the differences in feeding habits and food requirements of the animals they select. It should be noted that some animals will not feed normally in captivity until they have become accustomed to their surroundings. Techniques of forced feeding may be required. On the other hand, cold-blooded animals may survive for long periods of time without feeding. Students will need to research this information carefully before making final decisions.

3. *Nutritional Value of Foods.* The importance of a balanced diet should be stressed. The teacher can review the

importance of proteins, carbohydrates, fats, minerals, and vitamins, to the normal function of the cell and organism. The liver's
role in converting glucose to fat or fat to glucose can be included.
Class members can provide suggestions for the main food groups
which can then be listed on the chalkboard. The list should
include: milk and related products; meat (including fish and
poultry); grains and starch-bearing vegetables; and, finally, fruits
and vegetables. *Which of the materials essential to the body would
each group provide?*

Some home economics students might be familiar with the
complete (meat, milk, fish, eggs, cheese) and incomplete (peas,
beans, lentils, soybeans, peanuts) proteins, and might also be able
to explain that their "completeness" depends upon whether they
provide all the amino acids we need. They can use this list as a
help in identifying the materials the various groups provide.
Library research will help suggest the sources of carbohydrates,
fats, proteins, minerals, and vitamins.

Here again the teacher can stress that our location on the
food chain levels indicates the efficiency of the system, so that
a man depending on plants for his food, gets more energy per
pound of food than a man depending on animals for food.

If the teacher wishes, the class might prepare a display of
information gathered and can also include some lists of specific
foods of other cultures and countries, showing where they fit in
the food groups. An advanced class might also attempt to evaluate
such a diet as to how effectively it provides all nutritional needs.
The local hospital can arrange for a trip through its diet kitchen
and provide for a lecture by the dietician explaining the significance of the special diets prepared for those suffering various
illnesses.

4. *What Factors Limit Food Production?*   A class-developed
list would serve as an ideal review for all of the environmental
dangers previously covered in earlier lessons, including the problems of the availability of raw materials, sunlight, and space. Once
again students are faced with the cycle of increased population,
increased demands, and less space and materials to meet these
demands.

A very worthwhile reading assignment which could lead into
a discussion neatly summarizing the lesson can be found in chapter

5 of *Population, Resources, Environment,* by Paul and Ann Ehrlich.

5. *New Sources of Food.* Some consideration should be given to new sources of food and new ways to increase productivity. Students chould contact the Food and Agriculture Organization of the United Nations or the International Agricultural Development Service of the United States Department of Agriculture for information concerning increased yields of crops. These groups will provide them with information on new farming techniques as well as new strains of crops.

Students have no doubt heard a great deal about the possibility of using plants from the sea as an important source of food. It should be pointed out that seaweed, for example, as a major staple of many Asian diets, is now being considered as a food source for the western world. Students should be encouraged to connect concepts developed in previous lessons. For example, what connection does water pollution have to "harvesting" the sea? *What about overdoing it?* This point should be stressed over and over again. Unless we can restrain nations, commercial enterprises, and even individuals, any possible food sources are likely to be harvested at such a rapid rate that they would not be able to reproduce themselves.

The class can be asked to list plants and animals which serve as sources of food. *What about simple plant life?* A great deal of information dealing with research into single cell and protein food sources is available. Students might even culture some of these in class. Chlorella, for example, may be obtained from supply houses and can be used to investigate growth rate, culture requirements, and related information by setting up simple, student-designed experiments.

What Can You Do?

1. Make it a habit to eat a well-balanced diet. Do not push aside the salad or vegetable portion of your meals.
2. Use vegetable skins. Most of the vitamins in vegetables and fruits are in the skins. So do not waste them. Eat them.

3. You should diversify your diet. Do not always stick to "meat and potatoes."
4. Check your diet carefully to make certain it is a well-balanced one.

Pertinent Facts

1. Green plants are the only organisms which can manufacture food from raw materials.
2. There may be four or more levels in a food chain, with substantial energy loss at each level.
3. Proteins, carbohydrates, fats, vitamins, and minerals are all essential to proper body function.
4. Soil quality, weather conditions, and a host of other factors limit food production.

Possible Quiz

1. Using man as a carnivore, develop a hypothetical food chain identifying producers and various consumers.
2. Explain why man as a secondary consumer uses less food than man as a tertiary consumer.
3. Identify the four basic food groups, give an example of each, and identify the needed substances that each group provides.
4. Identify some of the factors which limit food production and availability.
5. What do we mean by food consumption—diminishing returns?

READINGS

Baker, B., and H. Kotsonis, *Modern Lesson Plans for the Biology Teacher.* West Nyack, N.Y., Parker Publishing Co., Inc., 1970.

Borgstrom, Georg, *Too Many.* Toronto: Collier-Macmillan, 1969.

Ehrlich, Paul, and Anne Ehrlich, *Population, Resources, Environment.* San Francisco: W.H. Freeman and Co., 1970.

Hendricks, Sterling, *Resources and Man.* San Francisco: W.H. Freeman and Co., 1969.

FILMS

"Marine Ecology." 29 minutes, sound, color, $8.15. McGraw-Hill Book Co., Text-Film Division, 330 West 42nd Street, N.Y., N.Y. 10018.

Urban Ecology

UNIT 4

LESSON 15

Rodents and Insects

Lesson time: 45-90 minutes

Aim

To examine, through the use of films and case studies, the effects of increased urbanization on the problems of rodent and insect infestation together with a look at the processes by which control is attempted.

Materials

films

Planned Lesson

1. *Rats.* The film, "Rats," is an excellent introductory film to spark discussion of the rat problem in urban areas. This film reviews ways in which rats enter buildings, feed, reproduce, do damage and can be controlled. The teacher might wish to spend added time reviewing the film material. Using the film's information on rats as a point of reference, students can identify ways in which rats enter buildings. Holes in walls, burrows, overhead wires, and other entries should be considered. They might conduct a survey of their own homes or the school building. *How can such*

entries be eliminated? Why is it important to eliminate trash around buildings? This can serve as a basis for a discussion of material on rat lodging. *If rats have no material with which to establish their home, will this help in their control?*

What do rats eat? Here it is important to stress that rats must always be chewing even if not eating due to the continuous growth of their front teeth. This growth ranges from three to six inches a year. The group can go on to consider the kind of foods that rats eat, much of it inadvertently provided by man. It should be clear that leaving food on the table in dirty dishes or in a sink is, in effect, providing a meal for possible pests. Open garbage pails, dumps containing food materials, or crumbs on the floor might be listed as well. Some students can research the millions of dollars of damage done each year by rats. The eating of stored grain, food crops, and other agriculture related damage might be considered also. *Why is it important to use closed metal garbage cans?* The need for closed cans should be obvious, but why not plastic garbage bags for example? Because rats can and do chew through plastic, it would be unwise to use plastic bags alone as containers unless the garbage was going to be collected very soon after being bagged. This makes it impractical.

The teacher can mention that rodent control programs generally leave poisoned food matter in sealed plastic bags to protect it from rain and other factors. The rats simply chew through the plastic. This can lead to a discussion of the kinds of materials used as poisons and the foods in which they might be placed. It should be noted that rats sense and therefore do not eat some kinds of poison. The poison commonly used in control programs is warfarin which is not poisonous to human beings or pets. This substance is frequently mixed with corn meal, an acceptable food to the rats. The class could research the various techniques used by exterminators for preparing food and placing it for likely consumption. This will vary with the specific area being studied. Rats may be found in sewer systems, buildings, food stores, construction sites, fields of growing crops, and a great many other locations.

Does your community have a rat control program? Usually such programs have an educator or public information staff which is anxious to come into the schools as a way of educating youngsters about the problem and indirectly educating their families. They can provide a speaker, films, and samples of traps, food bags, and the various pieces of equipment they use. Classes always seem to be very enthusiastic about the lectures.

2. *What Damage Do Rats Do and What Diseases Do They Cause?* Moving from the damage to crops and stored food supplies, the class can go on to a discussion of the diseases which rats might carry. Plague, typhus, leptospirosis, and toxoplasmosis can serve as the basis for this study. The teacher could also include here a brief lecture on zoonoses in general, explaining that they are diseases of animals which are transmitted to man. (Perhaps a student will note that this ability to transmit to man is what makes disease research on animals meaningful.) The list of well-known zoonoses, including those of animals other than rats might include diphtheria, encephalitis, parrot fever, tuberculosis, ringworm, tapeworm, trichinosis, and a host of others. This can be developed into a detailed discussion considering causative agent and host, or might just be a brief note identifying the term "zoonosis" and providing a few examples. In the case of rat zoonoses, students should determine the causative agent which is generally the flea.

Rat bite must also be included in the list of damages. Most Board of Health offices of large cities indicate that few rat bites are reported but that they are known to be common in areas of rat infestation. *Why do rats bite?* The teacher may prefer to omit the discussion of why rats bite since they suggest the horrid results such bites may have. Yet, the very seriousness of the problem is brought home by such topics. It will be necessary to consider the individual class in this matter. If the teacher explores the question, it will be important to note that rats eat bits of human tissue which they bite off, but may also bite because they are trying to eat food on that tissue. Unfortunately, this is not uncommon in the case of babies in cribs who have been given a bottle. The milk on the child's face attracts the rat. This can be connected with leprosy as well, since it was long thought that the loss of fingers, toes, and nose tips was due to the disease. It was later determined that the disease caused a lack of sensation and that, actually, the tissue was lost to rats while the sleeping lepers were unable to feel the pain involved. It might be added here that directly or indirectly rats are responsible for about 50,000 deaths a year.

Chewing on electrical wires is another serious form of damage done by rats because this produces short circuits and causes fires. Large numbers of fires in older buildings particularly, are traced to rats. Students will easily locate information on this by reading newspaper articles, contacting local fire departments, or obtaining material from local, state, or federal rodent control programs.

3. *What About Insect Infestation?* A list of insects associated with household infestation should be developed. Cockroaches, termites, ants, bedbugs, wasps, hornets, and bees can be included. Other insects indigenous to the local area should be identified as well. The ways in which these pests do harm should be explored. Perhaps an individual or group could report on the biology of each insect's life cycle and habits.

4. *What Do Insects Eat?* It should be emphasized that a number of common household practices provide food for insects. *What kind of things are done in the home which might encourage insect infestation?* Here, the teacher will find that a few suggestions will elicit a long list of responses. These include leaving food crumbs on the table or floor, allowing pet dishes or other containers to fill with water and remain stagnant, putting bread crumbs out for the birds, allowing food or food scraps to remain uncovered, and not keeping garbage in properly closed containers.

5. *How Can We Get Rid of Insects?* Students should be warned about the careless use of commercial insecticides. If it has not been assigned earlier, this would be a good point at which to discuss Rachel Carson's *Silent Spring*. The need to understand the dangers to self and environment must be stressed. *How can we safely use commercial insecticides?* This can be developed from the earlier lessons. The group might also want to contact the county agricultural agent to arrange for a visit and/or a lecture to the class. The discussion should also consider when a professional exterminator should be used.

The teacher can show the interrelationships which have come to the fore during the discussions. It should be noted that insect and rodent infestations can be avoided by taking precautions against providing them food and by alert and constant efforts of all involved. The topic can conclude with some consideration of the tremendous problems facing irradication programs in large cities. Aspects of this include public education, adequate garbage collection service, the need for everyone to cooperate, problems of buildings which provide entries for pests, and the need for massive irradication programs.

A strong conclusion can be developed by presenting the class with information concerning rat reproduction. There are several types of rats which contribute to the infestation problem, but generally we can say that rats mature in about five months and then begin producing litters of from five to eighteen young. They can have another litter within a few months. If, for example, the teacher asks the class to determine the number of rats which would result from the union of just one male and one female rat at the end of a year, the impact of the problem will be obvious to all. This can be taken a step further by computing the total family size assuming that half of each litter is male and half female, and that all interbreed every three months to produce a litter of twelve. Even if the class assumes that a given percentage do not survive or reproduce, the numbers will be impressive. The lesson can end with a discussion of federal pest control programs, the problems they might face, and the results if a control program were suddenly stopped. A final question to ponder: Can we eradicate such pests or can we even control them?

What Can You Do?

1. Conduct a survey of your home or of your school building. If you discover holes in walls or burrows, have them eliminated. This will prevent the entry of rats and other animals.
2. Eliminate trash from around the school building or your home. Keep all such trash covered with a tight lid.
3. Do not leave food on the table, in dirty dishes, or in a sink. This will only serve to provide food for a variety of pests.
4. If your community does not have one, organize a campaign to set up a rat control program.
5. Similar programs should also be established for insect control.
6. Leaving crumbs on the floor or table, or around the

outside of your home for birds, can serve as an attractant for a variety of insect pests.

Pertinent Facts

1. Rats enter buildings through holes in walls, broken windows, and other entries and use rubbish as a shelter.
2. Control of rats generally involves preparing poisoned food with substances such as warfarin which causes internal bleeding and death.
3. Rats carry disease, destroy crops and stored food, bite and may even kill human beings.
4. Insects carry disease, destroy food and materials of various kinds, cause painful and occasionally fatal bites, and are a nuisance.
5. Both rats and insects breed when carelessness provides food for them. Garbage, dropped food scraps, stagnant water, and similar sources all provide food or breeding sites for them.
6. Pest infestation is a serious urban problem demanding a multifaceted and large-scale attack.

Possible Quiz

1. Identify five things you could do to make an urban dwelling "rat proof."
2. List and discuss three ways in which rats do damage.
3. Compare the steps you would follow to reduce possible rat infestation with those for insect control. Why are urban control groups set up for both rat and insect work?
4. What are some pesticides that you could use safely to control insects?
5. The difficulties of both rodent and insect control are closely involved with the rate of reproduction of each and the adaptations of each. Identify and discuss four aspects of this.

READINGS

Carson, Rachel, *Silent Spring.* Boston: Houghton-Mifflin, 1962.

Elton, Charles S., *The Ecology of Invasions by Animals and Plants.* New York: Wiley, 1958.

Langer, William L., "The Black Death," *Scientific American.* Vol. 210, No. 2, February, 1964.

Steele, James H., *Animal Disease and Human Health,* Basic Food Study No. 3. Rome: United Nations Food and Agricultural Organization, 1962.

FILMS

"Listen to the Rat Man." Color, sound, 24 minutes. Environmental Health Service, U.S. Department of Health, Education, and Welfare, Washington, D.C.

"Rats." Sound, color, 32 minutes. UCOM Educational, Inc., 907 Culver Road, Rochester, N.Y. 14609

LESSON 16

Waste Disposal

Lesson time: **90 minutes**

Aim

To investigate the kinds of wastes generated by large megalopolises, and to examine the problems caused by the need to dispose of these wastes.

Materials

films

Planned Lesson

In the study of rodent and insect control, the proper disposal of waste was seen as a crucially important aspect of any program. Using this as a point of reference, the teacher can begin to develop the entire subject of waste disposal.

1. *What Kinds of Waste Do We Generate?* A long list of different kinds of waste can be developed ranging from construction materials to dead animals and including human and animal feces, combustibles such as boxes, clothing, and garden clippings, cans, furniture, glass, discarded appliances, and a-bandoned automobiles. Although the amount of matter can be compared to population increases, some consideration should also

131

be given to our changing society which provides a wider and wider range of materials for our use. It should also be pointed out that we have been moving toward a "throw-away" society with all the related difficulties such as the ultimate disposal of nonreturnable containers and synthetic materials. In the past, the smaller quantities of waste materials were composed of more easily degradable substances.

2. *What Do Cities Do with Garbage?* The term garbage can be used to cover all the various solid wastes. Students should establish a committee to study local waste disposal, and perhaps arrange for a field trip and guest speaker. (Communities which use incinerators may not allow visitors because of high temperatures and the risk of injury.)

The study of garbage disposal should include open dumpings in which piles of garbage simply build up on specified sites. *What problems have you studied which would be intensified by such dumping?* If the community has open dumping, some research can be done to determine whether any insect or rodent controls are used. Students should also investigate the problem of spontaneous fires. This common problem will be known to them because the summer fires cause clouds of smoke and bad odors which may last for days. Using some review of microbial action, it can be explained that the decaying of the garbage is a process during which microbes release heat. The total amount in a pile of garbage may be enough to reach the kindling temperature of the garbage and the fire begins. Because dumps are usually large and without water supplies, the fires are hard to control.

Sanitary landfill sites are also used quite extensively. *How do they differ from open dumping?* Here the idea is to cover the garbage with soil so that rats cannot get to it, insect eggs cannot hatch in it, and fires can be avoided. This method, of which several variations may be used, is more expensive since it requires careful planning and therefore trained people. The problems connected with this method also include the contamination of ground water, as rain passes through it and down into the water table.

A discussion of incinerators can be used to illustrate that they efficiently reduce large quantities of garbage to small amounts of ash and tiny particles. By reviewing the lesson on air pollution, however, students can see that such incinerators substantially add to the particles in the air. Afterburners on incinerators may solve the problem. It should be quite evident that the problem of nonburnable wastes cannot be solved by incineration.

It should also be noted that composting is being tried as a method of disposing of organic materials. Long of interest to some gardeners and farmers, the use of composting has increased in popularity and has attracted much attention as will be seen in Lesson 17, Organic Gardening. Large-scale composting has been and is successfully used in many countries. It simply involves the shredding of organic matter and its decay by microbes so that compost or decayed matter is produced. It is then used to enrich the soil. On a large scale some obvious problems will be evident. Nondecaying materials such as metals and plastic must be removed before composting begins, and they must then be disposed of by some other means. *How is compost used?* Students will probably indicate that it is used to improve soil, may be sold or even given free to farmers and gardeners, and is used by local parks and other recreational areas.

3. *What About Collection Campaigns?* An excellent class project could develop from a collection campaign for bottles, cans, or newspapers. Bottle and can return centers are proliferating at great speed and are widely advertised. A committee of the entire class can be set up to investigate first the need for such a project, and then the means by which to accomplish it. They might find that paper collection is already being done as this has long been one of the few financially feasible materials to collect for recycling. It would be interesting for them to research the subject in order to determine how many bottles and cans, how much paper, or whatever else they choose to work on, is discarded each year in the United States (55 billion cans, 26 billion jars and bottles, 65 billion bottle caps, 7 million cars). Such a project will provide not only actual activity in improving the environment, but will also give experience in organizing a complex, multi-faceted project. The group can contact virtually any company which uses glass or metal containers for their products in order to locate nearby collection centers. Wastepaper dealers can be located in the local telephone directory. Students will have to deal with collection

procedures, special preparations (such as removing metal from bottles or tying paper), publicity, and a great many other details which will help them to develop responsibility and a sense of organization. They should also check on the existence of other groups already involved in such projects. It may be wiser to join an existing campaign than to have students develop one on their own.

4. *What About Sewage Treatment?* Human wastes are certainly also a part of our waste disposal problem. An interested student might report on the history of sewage disposal, citing perhaps the disease epidemics connected with the lack of such disposal. It should also be noted that sewage also includes any other wastes which are emptied into the sewage system, such as wastes from industrial processes. The group should consider the treatment of sewage and in preparation should know that engineers measure sewage in terms of organic particles suspended in water. These proteins, fats, and carbohydrates compose only one-half of one percent of the sewage, but they may represent hundreds of tons per day in a major city. The remaining 99.5 percent of sewage is water.

The teacher should review with the class the steps in the process of treatment in a sewage plant. These should include passage from the home into the sewage system, where, as it moves along, microbes begin degrading organic matter. A description of the plant itself should include screening to remove large objects, the settling of heavy particles in special chambers or tanks, treatment by filtering, aeration, or other techniques to chemically stabilize effluent, and final settling and chlorination. It should be mentioned that original settling is known as primary treatment, whereas filtering, aeration, and similar processes are secondary treatment. At this point reference can be made to Lesson 1—Water Pollution, to connect sewage treatment to the pollution problem. It is quite likely that students have read articles on the need for tertiary treatment. The discussion in Lesson 1 on population increase and taxed sewage plants can be the focus for the study. Students should investigate procedures in their own communities. The local sewage treatment plants can usually be visited as a field trip experience. In some cases they may even be temporarily shut down to allow for a less odoriferous tour, but there are two negative aspects to such a shutdown. First of all, it may be impossible to shut down the plant which must operate continuously just to keep pace with sewage volume. This seems to be universally true in cities where plant capacity is always taxed. Secondly, a study of ecology should be an honest one. Students are frequently very enthusiastic and seem to be extremely interested in various ecological problems as long as they can be comfortable about it. The moment some actual labor or any unpleasantness is involved, the teacher will be able to determine which students are really maturely involved. A trip to an operating sewage plant is likely to be such an experience. It is important that students get to see the realities including the fact that real people work in unpleasant surroundings. As a result similar experiences or even films will tend to make the problems "real" and "immediate."

Whether their community uses them or not, all types of sewage systems should be studied since it is important that classes understand that pollution is not a local problem, but is one that must be considered on the basis of all the biological cycles. The water cycle, for example, may ultimately carry the water we use today to other areas of the globe.

Cesspools, for example, are just holes into which waste is poured. Ultimately bacteria of the soil break down or degrade this waste but it may also contaminate the water table. Septic tanks are somewhat more complex involving tile pipe which carries liquid from a water retention box or septic tank, to a field in which the liquid percolates through the soil and its contents degrade. The greater amount of solid waste settles in the tank which must be periodically emptied. Microbial action is depended on to degrade the wastes. Again water pollution can and does occur here. Also, careful engineering is required for the system to operate properly.

5. *The Relation of Sewage Disposal to Water Pollution.* Lesson 1 discusses oxygen depletion and water pollution. Here the point might be stressed again from the aspect of the microbial degradation of waste. Microbes require oxygen for the digestion process and therefore, students can surmise that effluent containing untreated or partially-treated waste causes a loss of oxygen in a

stream or river as microbes use it to digest the organic matter. The term "biodegradable" should be now understood by the class. The teacher may wish to explain that some detergents do not get broken down by microbes, might interfere with treatment plant operation, and ultimately come foaming out of the faucet. These nondegradable detergents have been now replaced with those that are biodegradable. The phosphate problem can be related to the oxygen problem by pointing out that some small plant life, like algae, thrive on phosphates and therefore use up too much of the available oxygen. Obviously treatment plants cannot filter out phosphates.

What Can You Do?

1. Set up a collection campaign for cans, bottles, or newspapers.
2. Call local scrap metal or salvage companies to see if they will purchase the cans you collect.
3. You can contact the Glass Container Manufacturers Institute, 330 Madison Avenue, New York, N.Y. 10017, to learn more about their glass reclamation program. They will pay ½¢ for each glass bottle or jar that is returned to them.
4. Do not throw your old jars or bottles away. Re-use them. They are ideal for storing a variety of items.
5. Save and bundle your old newspapers and magazines. Check your community to see if it has established reclamation centers for these items. If none exist, perhaps you can start one as a school project.
6. Have your parents and friends establish the practice of separating their trash into cans, bottles, wet garbage, and paper.

Pertinent Facts

1. Today we generate greater quantities of waste then ever before, and waste which is harder to dispose of because

of its chemical makeup and the limits of space and technology.

2. Dumps, incinerators, and composting are all means for disposing of wastes, but each of these has unique drawbacks.

3. Sewage is a major part of our waste disposal problem which may also contribute to water pollution.

4. Some sewage is dumped into waterways with little or no treatment, although in many cases tertiary treatment is needed to produce a nonpolluting effluent.

5. Cesspools and septic tanks are forms of waste disposal which are usually less adequate than municipal systems since they frequently cause pollution of the water table.

Possible Quiz

1. What kinds of facilities does your community have for garbage disposal? Explain how they operate.

2. Describe the local methods of sewage treatment. (If this is a sewage plant, the teacher might also ask, "What body of water does the effluent enter? Is the effluent completely degraded at the plant?")

3. How effective is recycling in your community?

4. Each method of garbage disposal has related problems. Discuss them.

5. How does sewage treatment affect the purity of the waterway the effluent enters?

READINGS

Ehlers, V.M. and E.W. Steel, *Municipal and Rural Sanitation.* New York: McGraw-Hill and Company Inc., 1965.

Gross, Edward, "Digging Out From Under," *Science News.* Vol. 96, 1969.

Herber, Lewis, *Crisis in Our Cities.* Englewood Cliffs, New Jersey: Prentice-Hall, Inc., 1968.

FILMS

"Forest Murmurs: The Problem of Litter." 9 minutes, sound, color, $4.00. University of Michigan, Audio-Visual Education Center, 416 Fourth Street, Ann Arbor, Michigan 48103.

"Good Riddance," 25 minutes, color, sound, $8.00. University of Michigan.

"Up to Our Necks." 26 minutes, color, sound, $14.40. NBC Educational Enterprises, 30 Rockefeller Plaza, Room 914, New York N.Y. 10022.

LESSON 17

Organic Gardening

Lesson time: 45 minutes

Aim

To implement the concept of recycling through preparation and observation of decay in a compost pile, and to appreciate the advantages and disadvantages to man and the environment of organic gardening.

Materials

> twigs
> grass cuttings
> leaves
> cans

Planned Lesson

1. *What Is an Organic Food?* The student should not confuse the chemical definition of organic and inorganic here. The discussion should be so directed so that they will come to understand that organic foods are those which are grown without artificial help of any kind. *What substances would not be permitted? In relation to early studies, how would this affect various pollution problems?*

2. *How Is Organic Farming and Gardening Done?* The various problems of farming should be listed and possible methods of solution suggested. For example, insect infestations may be eliminated by using insecticides or by introducing natural enemies such as praying mantises. Poor soil may be improved with chemical fertilizers or a compost heap may be started to provide decayed vegetable matter. Animals may be fed antibiotics, vaccines, or other chemicals, or they may receive a nutritious balanced organic diet. Food processing, when necessary, can be done with or without chemicals.

A valuable and educational experience for students is the establishment and study of a compost heap. The class should first plan an inconspicuous location for the heap and then get appropriate permission for its development. They can then organize into groups to collect material from the school grounds, prepare the heap, and add to it. The project also helps to develop an interest in improving the appearance of the environment. The pile will include grass cuttings (try to plan the first work on the day that the grass will be cut), twigs, dead leaves, perhaps scraps of paper, wood, cans, and other debris. The pile should be covered over with soil, especially if it contains any material which serves as food for pests like rats. If the material is exclusively garden debris and is turned throughly every few days or so, it may decompose within a few weeks (depending on the local climate). The teacher may prefer to leave it undisturbed (except for additions) for a long period of time, after which it can be spread out throughly and the rate of decay studied. *Did all materials decompose? Which did not?*

3. *Advantages of Organic Gardening and Farming.* Points to be stressed would include a large scale reduction in the use of pesticides, the decreasing resultant health hazard and water and soil pollution; the elimination of chemicals, including DDT, from the human diet; recovery of valuable organic matter for the soil; reduction in the volume of waste to be disposed of; and better quality soil and foods. A survey of the amount of organic matter disposed of in the average home will surprise the students. They should survey their own homes and observe the disposal of vegetables and fruit peelings, stale food and bread and other organic matter. Perhaps, if the family cooperates, a separate

garbage can can be used to collect a few days' accumulation of organic garbage. Virtually every household can produce compost and return needed material to the soil.

4. *Is Organic Gardening a Fad?* Student opinions on the value of eating chemical-free fruit should be sought. *What disadvantages are there to organic gardening?* If students consider each characteristic they will realize that some fruit is likely to contain worms, that the lack of chemical supplements may mean somewhat smaller fruit, and that lack of preservatives means that foods will spoil faster. However, they will also see that they will not be ingesting chemicals which may be harmful, the foods they eat will not have the taste altered by chemicals, and the foods will probably taste better because they will not be picked before ripening and then preserved. These factors, together with the ecological advantages of recycling waste and the improvement of the soil, should help students to see that the basic principles of organic gardening are sound. For further information students should seek out a nearby organic gardening club.

What Can You Do?

1. As part of a school project, establish an organic garden on the school grounds. See how many different kinds of fruits and vegetables you can grow without the use of pesticides.
2. Establish a compost heap in your backyard. Instead of burning your grass and leaf cuttings, simply add them to this heap.
3. Conduct a survey of your home and determine the amount of organic matter disposed of. This can be added to your compost heap instead of being thrown out as "garbage."

Pertinent Facts

1. Organic foods are those raised without artificial help.
2. Organic gardeners use natural predators to control insects and compost to improve soil.

3. Composting helps to dispose of waste and helps to improve the quality of the soil.
4. The practices of organic gardening help to reduce pollution.
5. Organic gardening is an ancient method which has become popular as a result of concern for the condition of the environment.

Possible Quiz

1. What substances commonly used by farmers and gardeners would not be used in organic methods?
2. How do organic gardeners cope with common garden problems?
3. How do you build a compost heap and what does it do?
4. In what ways does organic gardening help to improve the environment?
5. What are some disadvantages of organic gardening?

READINGS

Davis, Adelle, *Let's Cook It Right.* Pittsburgh, Pennsylvania: Natural Sales Co., 1971.

Rodale, Robert, *The Basic Book of Organic Gardening.* Emmaus, Pennsylvania: Rodale Press, 1971.

Organic Gardening and Farming Magazine is a monthly periodical devoted to this topic. It is published by Rodale Press Inc., Emmaus, Pennsylvania, 18049.

FILMS

"Birth of the Soil." 10 minutes, sound, color, $3.00. Visual Instruction Service, I.S.U., Ames, Iowa 50010.

"Our Soil Resources." 10 minutes, sound, black and white, $1.65. Visual Instruction Service.

LESSON 18

Cause and Effect
of Malnutrition

Lesson time: 45 minutes
Laboratory time: 90 minutes

Aim

To utilize knowledge of nutrition in planning well-balanced meals and to understand the symptoms and physiological damage of malnutrition.

Materials

iodine	samples of basic food groups
Benedict's solution	reducing sugar
Sudan III	indophenol
silver nitrate	ninhydrin solution
citrus juice	test tubes
test tube holders	

Planned Lesson

1. *What Are the Requirements for Good Nutrition?* The study of malnutrition must be based on a solid understanding of good nutrition. The lesson might begin with a class attempt at developing the requirements of good nutrition. Fortunately there

143

has been a resurgence of interest on the part of food processors and government agencies in establishing public education campaigns on good nutrition. Students will therefore have been exposed to some information dealing with human nutritional requirements, and should be able to identify the four food groups. A chalkboard list would include: milk and dairy products; meat, eggs, poultry; grains, potatoes and other related vegetables; fruit, and leafy green and yellow vegetables.

Examples of each category can be included and, if the teacher feels it advisable, students might call upon their knowledge of cell physiology to identify which foods provide the basic substances (including vitamins, minerals, fat, protein, and carbohydrates). Such a review would be very valuable as a prelude to studying some of the specific problems of malnutrition. Assigning student oral reports on the various cell substances is one device for developing a knowledge of their importance.

If time permits and it is deemed worthwhile, the following laboratory activity can be used here. Have students test various common foods of their choice for the presence of carbohydrates, fat, and protein. The presence of vitamin C and chloride ions can also be tested. They can use a few drops of iodine on a starchy food (bread, cake, potato) to identify the characteristic blue-black color; Benedict's solution, mixed and heated with a reducing sugar for the yellow-green to brick red color change; Sudan III on a peanut or other fatty substance to identify its absorption; indophenol with citrus juice to observe the characteristic color change; silver nitrate solution with a food containing a chloride for the characteristic silver chloride precipitate; and ninhydrin solution for the characteristic purple color when heated with a protein. Students should be cautioned to heat test tubes carefully, hold them with appropriate holders, and always make sure that the mouth of the tube *does not* point toward anyone. (The ninhydrin test requires a fresh solution in order to be successful.)

2. *How Widespread Is Malnutrition?* Students should be asked to estimate the percentage of the world population which is malnourished. Their estimates will usually reflect the fact that they live in a society in which most people are believed to be

adequately fed. They may be startled to discover that only about one-sixth of the world's population can be described as being adequately fed. Even more surprising, a large segment of the American population is as malnourished as the people of many underdeveloped countries.

Some consideration must be given to the interrelationships of increased population and hunger. *Why are famines due to floods, wars, or other disasters different from those due to increased population? What are some environmental factors which contribute to malnutrition?*

3. *Deficiency Diseases.*   Student reports can present material on the various deficiency diseases including rickets, osteomalacia, beriberi, night-blindness, kwashiorkor, scurvy, and pellagra. It should be stressed that these are not limited to other countries or even poor areas of our country. Many pediatricians report having treated rickets, for example, due to Vitamin D deficiency. The practice of giving cod liver oil or synthetic vitamin preparations to infants and children is fairly common and should be introduced as usual today. Interested students might want to consult *Scientific American,* December, 1970, for the article on Vitamin D.

What are the results of malnutrition? The range of effects of malnutrition include lowered resistance to disease, physical deformities in children, brain damage in children, emotional and mental disorders in adults, and death. The lesson provides for an excellent review and integration of ideas and concepts presented in earlier lessons.

What Can You Do?

1. Try to eat a balanced meal as often as possible. Eat your salad and fruit as well as your meat and vegetables.
2. Do not throw leftovers away. You can eat them the next day, or they can be used to enhance the diet of your pet.
3. Save the scraps from your meals and add them to your organic garden or compost heap. If you do not have one, start one.

Pertinent Facts

1. Malnutrition is a state of life for most of the world's population.
2. Proper nutrition provides for adequate amounts of foods, vitamins, and minerals in the daily diet.
3. Famines due to increased population size are of particular concern because they are not temporary as are those due to a disaster.
4. A number of deficiency diseases caused by malnutrition exist, and contribute to body damage.
5. Many ecological factors combine to produce famine and malnutrition.

Possible Quiz

1. Identify the main food groups, listing two examples of foods in each and telling what materials they provide.
2. List four deficiency diseases, give their causes, and symptoms.
3. Identify five effects of malnutrition on the human body.
4. Discuss the implications of malnutrition on a society and its ability to overcome the problems it causes.

READINGS

Altman, Philip L. and Dorothy S. Dittmer (eds.), *Metabolism*. Bethesda, Maryland: Federation of American Societies for Experimental Biology, 1968.

Dumont, Rene and Bernard Rosier, *The Hungry Future*. New York: Praeger, 1969.

Paddock, William and Paul Paddock, *Hungry Nations*. Boston: Little, Brown, and Company, 1964.

FILMS

"Food Crisis." 60 minutes, sound, black and white, $12.00. Indiana University, A-V Center, Bloomington, Indiana 47401.

"Food for a Modern World." 22 minutes, sound, color, $7.50. University of Michigan, A-V Center, 416 Fourth Street, Ann Arbor, Michigan 48103.

"Food Revolution." 26 minutes, sound, color, $8.00. McGraw-Hill Text Films, 330 West 42nd Street, New York, N.Y. 10018.

LESSON 19

Sex Education
for the Student

Lesson time: 90 minutes
Laboratory time: 45 minutes

Aim

To provide the student with a thorough and basic understanding of the process by which human reproduction occurs,
from the development of egg and sperm to the birth of the new
organism.

Materials

> models of the male and
>   female reproductive
>   systems
> birth models
> films

Planned Lesson

This lesson might logically follow the study of the reproductive processes of lower species, or perhaps a series of lessons on
cell division and differentiation. If this is not the case, the teacher
should review the concepts of mitosis, meiosis, cleavage, and

differentiation. After such a review, it might be suggested that it would be interesting to follow these processes at work in the human being. The anatomy of the male and female reproductive system can then be introduced, organ by organ, as the study progresses. It has been our experience that if the subject is presented in a straightforward, relaxed manner, there will be little if any difficulties. The attitude of the student generally reflects that of the teacher, so that a relaxed, mature approach will elicit mature response.

1. *Anatomy of the Reproductive Tract.* Considering the general maturity of the class, the teacher may find it easier to use serial overhead transparencies which do not indicate any outline of the body until the final transparency in the serial. In this manner, the first transparency would illustrate only the ovaries, for example. The second transparency in the series would add the oviducts, and so on until the final overlay would indicate the outline of the body and the relative positions of these organs within the body. Ovaries in themselves do not evoke comments or jokes, and by the time the discussion is completed, most students have become so sincerely interested that the subject is no longer amusing. If overhead materials are not readily available, chalkboard sketches similar to Figure 19-1 will do as well, and can be developed in the same manner.

The teacher can then go on to a discussion of the general anatomy of the male reproductive tract in the same way. That is, by using a series of overlay transparencies and discussing the functions of the testes, epididymis, vas deferens, urethra, prostate, and penis, in a step-wise fashion.

2. *Formation of the Gametes.* Starting with the ovaries, a brief discussion should indicate their almond-like shape, location in the abdomen, and their function as a gonad, or structure which produces reproductive cells. *What reproductive cells, or gametes, do the ovaries produce? How does this occur?* The teacher may wish to consider this in some depth, or simply explain that females are born with a number of immature egg cells (approximately 40,000) deep within the ovaries, and that hormone levels of the blood with the onset of puberty trigger the egg to undergo meiosis as it slowly moves up to the surface of the ovary. As it reaches the

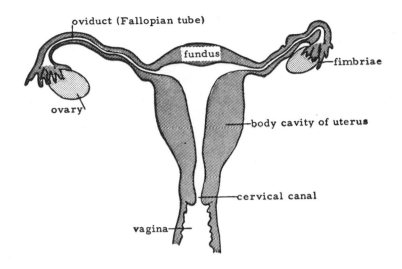

Figure 19-1. Female Reproductive System

surface of the ovary, a small pimple-like structure, the Graafian follicle, forms. Hormonal changes cause the follicle to rupture (ovulation) and release the egg. The ovulated egg then enters the oviduct (Fallopian tube) and continues down to the uterus.

At this point, the group will have to assume that the egg has not been fertilized, in which case it continues its travels and leaves the body through the vagina. If the group assumes that the egg has been fertilized, it would then be implanted in the lining of the uterus and would continue its development.

A word or two about the development of this lining and its elimination if fertilization does not occur will lead naturally into the concept of menstruation. Again the control by hormones should be stressed. It should also be noted that the lining is not sloughed off all at once, but rather in a precise pattern.

The release of this menstrual fluid will lead to a consideration of the hymen. It should be pointed out that this membrane across the cervical opening must normally have openings in it to allow for the menstrual flow. It should further be mentioned that the size of these openings vary from one individual to another, including those individuals who have virtually no membrane at all.

The formation of sperm can now be considered along parallel lines. The egg shape of the testes, and larger size as compared with the ovaries (25 gm as compared with 5-6 gm) should be noted, as well as the fact that they are located outside the body. The body temperature's effect on sperm should be explained in order to point out the need for the cooler temperature outside the body, in the scrotal sac. It should further be explained that, not only will sperm soon die at body temperature, but that they cannot be manufactured at that temperature.

The production of sperm by the seminiferous tubules of the testes (over 60 million sperm per ml of semen, or over a billion per ejaculation); its transfer to the epididymis for storage; its ultimate release by way of the urethra; and the accessory roles of the prostate gland, Cowper's glands, and the seminal vesicles should be discussed. *If only one sperm is needed to fertilize an egg, why are so many produced?* Here the role of hyaluronidase might be mentioned, as well as the concept of biological protection in providing insurance that the egg will be fertilized. It should also be noted that approximately half the sperm ejaculated will not be available for fertilization, since they will have moved into the second Fallopian tube (presumably the one in which no egg is present). Normally the ovaries alternate the process of ovulation so that one of the two Fallopian tubes will not have an egg in it at any one time.

3. *Fertilization.* In considering fertilization, students can refer to the concept of meiosis, as they realize that the egg and sperm are haploid, while the fertilized egg or zygote is diploid. Using Figure 19-1 of the female reproductive system, it can be illustrated that fertilization occurs in the oviduct when the egg has moved a short distance down its length. Fertilization, of course, requires that sperm be present. *How do the sperm move from the vagina through the uterus to the oviduct?* Sperm motility and the presence of a flagellum will be suggested by students. The teacher might mention that studies of human infertility problems are concerned with sperm motility as well as the total number of sperm produced.

4. *Development.* After fertilization, the zygote will require six to seven days to move down the oviduct and become implanted in the wall of the uterus. Early stages of development

need not be reviewed if cleavage and elementary embryology have recently been discussed. If the teacher wishes, Figure 19-2, illustrating early development and cleavage in the frog can be placed on the chalkboard for a quick review of these stages.

The teacher may wish to place the following outline on the chalkboard to indicate the various major developments occurring during pregnancy. Days are also numbered, with day 1 as the first day of the last menstrual period:

1. 13th day—fertilization
2. end of 3rd week (13th-22nd day)—ovum traveling down oviduct, floating in uterus
3. beginning 4th week (22nd day)—implantation; egg barely visible to the naked eye
4. beginning 5th week—minute grey-white flesh
5. end 5th week—backbone forming; 5-8 vertebrae; 1/12 of an inch long, 1/6 of an inch wide
6. beginning 6th week—head forming; heart visible
7. end 6th week—all backbone laid down; tail end of embryo distinct; beginnings of arms and legs visible; depressions where eyes will form; 1/4 of an inch long
8. 7th week—chest, abdomen formed; fingers and toes beginning; eyes visible; 1/2 inch long
9. 8th week—face, features forming; ears form; 7/8 of an inch long; weight—1/30 oz. (1 gram)
10. 9th week (end 2nd month)—face formed; arms, legs, hands, feet partly formed; stubby toes and fingers; 1-1/5 inches long; weight—1/15 oz.; looks like a miniature infant
11. end 3rd month (13-1/2 weeks)—nails appear; can determine sex; 3 inches long; weight—1 oz.; large head
12. end 4th month (18 weeks)—fetal movements; eyebrows and eyelashes; 8-1/2 inches long; weight—6 oz.
13. end 5th month (22-1/2 weeks)—hair on head; fat depositing; if born now may live a few hours at most; 8-1/2 inches long; weight—1 pound
14. end 6th month (27 weeks)—covered with vernix; skin wrinkled; eyes open; if born now one in ten may survive with expert care

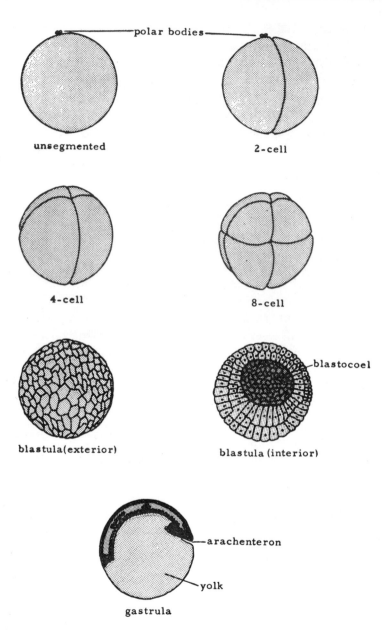

Figure 19-2. Stages of Cleavage and Early Development

15. end 7th month (31-1/2 weeks)—in male, testicles descend; 50% chance of surviving if born now; 16 inches long; weight—3 pounds.
16. end 8th month (35-3/4 weeks)—90% chance of surviving; 18 inches long; weight—5-1/4 pounds
17. end 9th month (40 weeks)—20 inches long; weight—7 pounds 6 ounces

It should be pointed out that the length of pregnancy is approximately 280 days from the first day of the last menstrual period. Approximately 4 percent of all babies are born on the 280th (due date) day; 54 percent are born before that date, and 42 percent after that date. A range of two weeks before to two weeks after the due date is considered the normal range in which the birth may occur.

A brief mention of the nature and function of the placenta should also be included. It is important that the class understand that the maternal and fetal blood never mix, but only circulate near each other as the capillaries of each are in close proximity in the placenta. *What passes between these two sets of capillaries? How?* Students may call upon past lessons on lung functioning, or the teacher may wish to explain the passage of molecules through the walls of the capillaries.

5. *Birth.* The birth process itself can be considered in three stages. If available, birth models and charts should be used. The first stage, or the beginning of labor, is usually first identified by irregularly-timed uterine contractions. The mucous plug which blocks the cervix may be released. This is the "bloody show." The membrane within the placenta, known as the amniotic sac, may rupture releasing the watery fluid which has cushioned the fetus. During this stage, the tissues over the cervix begin to get thin and then move back, so that the opening ultimately reaches a dilation of 10 cm. The contractions become very regular and can be precisely timed.

Now that the passage is cleared, what occurs in the second stage? Students will begin to realize that the fetus must now be moved down and out. Birth models or charts will help to show the movement in the usual head down and face to the mother's back position. Students should be encouraged to consider the likely contractions in the second stage. They will no doubt understand that these must be very powerful and close together in order to effect the actual birth.

The third stage, or delivery of the placenta, will occur a few minutes after the birth of the child, and usually occurs after one or two powerful uterine contractions. It should be emphasized that the uterus begins to contract immediately. This not only pushes out the placenta, or afterbirth, but also helps to constrict the blood vessels which rupture during the birth. This helps to prevent hemorrhage.

6. *Natural Childbirth.*   A word or two should be included about natural childbirth. The growing interest in being awake and aware during childbirth is reflected in an increasing number of questions on this method in the classroom. The most popular method of "natural childbirth" is actually a technique which came to the United States by way of a French doctor, Ferdinand Lamaze, and is more correctly known as the "Lamaze Method." This method depends upon special breathing techniques which help to relax muscles and thereby reduce discomfort due to uterine contractions. This also helps to block out nerve impulses of contractions to the brain. Although the method provides for anesthesia if requested by the mother, most women find that they need little or none. This method has proven very successful and is suggested by many obstetricians. Local and regional groups have been organized throughout the country, and will provide information and rent films on childbirth on request. (In the New York area the groups are generally known as the ASPO, or American Society for Psycho-Prophylaxis in Obstetrics.)

The Lamaze Method is considered advantageous because the child has not received any anesthetic (through the mother), the mother can speed the birth because she can voluntarily contract her muscles in assistance, and because the mother suffers no aftereffects of anesthesia, and can be ambulatory within a few hours after delivery.

Thus, the teacher can review the process of reproduction from meiosis and fertilization through birth by use of a film or several films. Particularly excellent ones are "The Sex Cells," "Fertilization," and "Naissance."

7. *Laboratory Activities.*   Laboratory time might be spent using film strips or films to emphasize the various concepts discussed during lecture. Students might also go to the library to research the topic, and might include famous names in medicine such as Semmelweis, or interesting questions as, *where* did the term Caesarian surgery come from?

Pertinent Facts

1. The gonads, or ovaries and testes, produce eggs (ova) and sperm, respectively, by means of the process known as meiosis.
2. Menstruation is the sloughing off of the uterine lining and indicates that an egg has not been fertilized or that a fertilized egg has not been implanted.
3. By the eighth week of development, the embryo resembles a human being.
4. The birth process involves a preparatory stage during which the cervix dilates, a second stage during which the fetus is delivered, and a final stage during which the placenta is expelled.
5. Natural childbirth involves the use of specially learned techniques of breathing and muscle control.

Possible Quiz

1. List the various organs of the male and female reproductive systems and indicate the functions of each.
2. Briefly explain the process of fertilization and implantation.
3. Explain the process by which an exchange of substances occurs between maternal and fetal blood.
4. Follow the passage of a fetus through the birth canal, indicating the major characteristics of each stage involved.

READINGS

Case, James F., and Vernon E. Stiers, *Biology: Observation and Concept.* New York: Macmillan Co., Inc., 1971.

Guyton, Arthur C., *Function of the Human Body.* Philadelphia: W.B. Saunders and Co., Inc., 1964.

Langley, L.L. and E. Cheraskin, *Physiology of Man.* New York: Reinhold Publishing Co., Inc., 1965.

Philleps, Edwin A., *Basic Ideas in Biology.* New York: Macmillan, 1971.

FILMS

"Naissance." 35 minutes, sound, black and white and color, $20. ASPO, West 91st Street, New York, New York, can provide information for local distributors.

"Reproduction, Growth, and Development: Fertilization." 21 minutes, sound, color, $8.15. McGraw-Hill Book Co., Text-Film Division, 330 West 42nd Street, New York, New York 10018.

"Reproduction, Growth, and Development: The Sex Cells." 17 minutes, sound, color, $8.15. McGraw-Hill Book Co., Text-Film Division.

LESSON 20

Fertility
and Infertility

Lesson time: 45-90 minutes

Aim

To investigate the various problems and conditions that might interfere with reproduction, and to provide information about dealing with the problem of infertility in man.

Materials

> guest speakers
> films

Planned Lesson

1. *What Conditions Might Interfere with Reproduction?* Following Lesson 19—Sex Education for the Student, the class will be prepared to discuss some of the conditions which might interfere with reproduction. Students might be asked to list points in the reproductive process at which fertilization can be prevented and the means by which it can be corrected. This will help to set the stage for the discussion.

Beginning with the ovaries, the immature eggs may never reach maturity. The cause for this might be hormonal, or perhaps the ovaries themselves are not present. *What could be responsible for this? Can it be corrected?* Students will probably be aware of the fact that hormone treatment is possible for a variety of problems, and such treatment might be possible in this situation. If ovaries did not develop properly or were surgically removed, the condition would be irreversible.

Moving along through each part of the reproductive tract, students could include a thick ovarian outer membrane which prevents ovulation; adhesions within the oviducts, which means that the walls will stick together preventing the passage of ova; inability of the egg to implant; improperly prepared uterine lining; inability of the uterus to retain a fetus; chemical imbalances in the uterus and vagina; uterine contractions which release the fetus too soon, and all the many other possibilities. The teacher should also mention that there are cases of infertility for which no explanation has been found. In the male, the problem of temperature will probably be mentioned first, since this was discussed in Lesson 19, as was the number and motility of sperm.

All of these cases of infertility can be researched by the students in current magazines as well as in texts and reference books. They should try to identify some of the cases which can be helped by surgery, as in the problem presented by a thick ovarian membrane as well as that of tubal adhesions. They should also try to identify cases where hormones might be used to treat the condition, as in irregular egg maturation and release (ovulation), implantation problems, and premature labor.

2. *Artificial Insemination.* Once they have considered the preceding problems, students can then go on to consider various other problems and their solution. Included should be a discussion of the process of artificial insemination, in which sperm may be used after it has been collected from the father, as in cases of motility problems or those in which the sperm count is low. (It should be pointed out that sperm can now be frozen and stored for long periods of time.) Sperm can also be obtained from an anonymous donor, matched for physical characteristics. It might be interesting to point out that wearing pants and tight undershorts has reduced, to some extent, the fertility of the human male, because this has increased the temperature of the testes.

If the teacher feels it would be advantageous, a local specialist in infertility or a gynecologist-obstetrician should be invited to the class for a question and answer session or a lecture. The name of such an individual can usually be obtained by contacting your local hospital.

3. *Current Advances.* The teacher may also want to include a discussion on current research into artificial wombs; "substitute" mothers who have someone else's fertilized egg implanted in her uterus; or the possibility of producing individuals from the body cells of another person.

Thus, it should be reviewed and emphasized that it is important for fertility to occur, that an egg be produced, that sperm be present in the oviduct at the same time the egg is present, and in sufficient numbers to fertilize the egg. It is also vital that the hormone balance be correct, that the physiology of the uterus be correct, and that the chemical environment of the cervix and vagina be conducive to sperm passage.

Pertinent Facts

1. Hormone balance, physical abnormalities, and chemical imbalances are some of the factors responsible for infertility.
2. Infertility may be treated by surgery or with hormone therapy.
3. In cases where chemical or surgical therapy is not indicated, artificial insemination may be successful.

Possible Quiz

1. What alterations in the reproductive cycle of the female could be caused by hormone imbalance? In the male?
2. What types of infertility might be treated surgically?
3. What are the common causes of infertility in the male?
4. What is artificial insemination? How can it be used to overcome infertility?

READINGS

Bishop, D.W., "Sperm Motility," *Physiological Review, 42:1,* 1962.

Carey, H.M., *Modern Trends in Human Reproductive Physiology.* London: Butterworth and Co., 1966.

Drell, V.A., *Oral Contraceptives.* New York: McGraw-Hill Book Co., Inc., 1968.

Guttmacher, Alan F., *Pregnancy and Birth.* New York: Signet Books, 1962.

Kleegman, S.J., and S.A. Kaufman, *Sterility.* Philadelphia: F.A. Davis and Co., 1965.

FILMS

"Reproduction, Growth, and Development: Reproductive Hormones." 24 minutes, sound, color, $8.15. McGraw-Hill Book Co., Text-Film Division, 330 West 42nd Street, New York, New York 10018.

LESSON 21

Overpopulation and
Population Control

Lesson time: 45 minutes

Aim

To examine the problems generated by an ever-increasing population on our natural resources, air, water, and land, and to consider the ways in which population increase may be controlled.

Materials

films

Planned Lesson

1. *Overpopulation.* With the current emphasis on ecological problems and their relationship to overpopulation, students will have some general background on the subject even before the lesson begins. They will have read and heard of the interrelationships of virtually all ecological difficulties with the problem of overpopulation. The teacher might provide some statistics as an introduction to the lesson. For example, the total human population of the earth was about five million in 8,000 B.C.; in about 30 A.D. estimates suggest that the population was about 250 million; in 1650 it was about 500 million; by 1850 it was one billion; and,

163

by 1930 it was two billion. *Has the population increased at a steady, constant rate? What factors might account for the population increase?* It might be advisable to have students prepare a graph showing the increase from 8,000 B.C. to the present. *Has the time needed for the population to double remained constant?*

After reviewing the problem of two people creating more than two additional people (two being their "replacements"), the concepts of birth rate (number of babies/1000 people/year) and death rate should be introduced. It has been estimated that if the world birth rate were to stabilize at two percent, the world population would double in about thirty-five years. *What factors have tended to increase or decrease birth rate?* This will require some consideration of the need for able-bodied hands to help farm the land and work around the home. The larger the family, the more help. Thus, children were an asset. As farm technology improved, and machines and chemical improvements were made, children were no longer an asset. They became a liability, and family size started to decrease. Students should research this on their own. They will find that the developed countries have smaller family units than underdeveloped countries. *How can this be explained? What factors affect the death rate?* Beginning with current society, the class could list the many medical advances which save the lives of newborn as well as unborn children, to those advances which greatly extend life.

Stress must also be placed on the interrelationship of pollution to the populations of developed countries. Because developed countries have such advanced technology, they use proportionally far more materials than underdeveloped nations. For example, the United States is responsible for using over one-fourth of the resources of the earth (and for producing the resultant pollution), although we represent far less than one-fourth of its total population. This is an important point which must be emphasized. (The United States birth rate is directly related to economic and educational levels. The highest birth rate in the United States is among the poorest, least educated families.)

The class might prepare individual lists of items they or their family might not have or services which would not be available to them if they lived in an underdeveloped nation. This provides an opportunity to consider the ways in which we add to pollution just in terms of our daily living.

2. *Should Something Be Done to Control Population?* Much of the current literature provides statistics which indicate that at current rates we will soon have "standing room only." And, if technology allows, we would soon overflow and over-populate the moon and near-by planets. Student committees might be organized to research this topic and report on current opinion and theories. *Will we be able to feed and support an ever-increasing population?*

3. *Population Control. What means could be used to slow population growth?* There are two points from which this problem may be attacked. It might logically begin with various forms of birth control. Students will probably be able to suggest that since contraception means the prevention of conception, methods will require that an egg or sperm do not meet, or that a zygote not be implanted.

Beginning with abstention and going through the rhythm method, condom, IUD, diaphragm, spermicidal creams, jellies, foams, douches, and contraceptive pills, the teacher could briefly explain the means by which each provides for contraception, and the likelihood of success for each. If it is not considered necessary to go into detail for each, discussion might center around the physiological aspects of keeping the cells apart or in preventing implantation.

These methods of contraception provide only temporary means, but there is also much publicity about the more permanent sterilization operations. *Which people are likely to request sterilization?* Television interviews, magazine articles, and other reports frequently involve people who have chosen salpingectomy or vasectomy. Generally, these are people who have completed their families and do not plan or wish to have more children. Salpingectomy involves removal of a portion of the oviducts, while vasectomy is the cutting and tying off of the vas deferens. It should be made clear to students that neither the oviducts nor vas deferens are involved in the production of hormones. Thus, the normal hormonal balance will still be maintained. *Since hormones are responsible for the characteristics of maleness and femaleness, does sterilization alter masculinity or femininity?*

This is an important point. When students understand that the operation merely blocks the passage of the cells, they will realize that the general fears of changes in sexuality have no basis in fact. It should also be noted that these operations are reversible to some extent (estimates vary), and that newer techniques are increasing the likelihood of reversibility.

The second possibility now available is abortion. A great many questions always arise concerning this topic. Because abortion laws and the controversy of changing them are so much a part of the news, it is important that accurate facts be provided. Students should know that abortion involves the removal of an already-imbedded zygote from the uterine wall, and that the timing of this removal is critical because of the developing placenta. As the embryo develops, its connections with the uterus through blood vessels increases, so that the possibility of hemorrhage increases as time goes by. Abortion is said to be safer than the delivery of a full-term fetus if performed by a physician *before* the twelfth week of pregnancy. Current popular literature frequently contains articles explaining the various techniques available. *Why are illegal abortions so dangerous?* Here the class should be able to provide such suggestions as the lack of skilled personnel involved, infection, hemorrhage, lack of proper equipment and facilities, and lack of drugs. It should be pointed out that forty-five percent of all maternal deaths in the United States are the result of illegal abortions. This is the single greatest cause of maternal death in America.

4. *What About the Future?* Such reported possibilities as pills for men, a "morning-after pill," a small metal rod chemically impregnated or injected under the skin, the great variety of new chemicals, and various new mechanical aids to sterilization surgery, would all provide excellent report topics.

The lesson might be concluded with a look at the possibility of some form of control beyond the individual. In a sense, the current concern about population is such a control as it influences individuals in a social way. Economic pressures to marry and have children are currently built into our tax laws (although there is no attempt to suggest that this was planned).

What methods could a government use to alter or control population growth? As a direct result of the preceding discussion, students will suggest tax laws to encourage smaller families. Adoption could also be encouraged. Students should be able to provide a long list of suggestions from the many public discussions going on around them. It is important to have them think through their suggestions thoroughly and carefully, in order to consider the ramifications. *Would penalizing a family financially benefit the children involved? How would that ultimately affect society?* The question of the government's "right" to control family size is always a controversial one. Some students believe it does not have such a right, while others feel it has as much right to limit the number of children as it does for the number of spouses one may have. Still others feel that they "can have them if they can support them," which is immediately countered with the idea that ultimately the question is "Can society support them?" It should be stressed that in March, 1971, a Presidential Commission did in fact suggest that the federal government begin to take steps in the area of population control. This would provide interesting report material as students research, report, and think through the many suggestions and the serious implications of each.

What Can You Do?

1. In terms of the current population "crisis," inform yourselves, as young adults, of the various birth control methods that are available. Also determine how effective these are.
2. Have your parents support birth control programs.
3. Have your parents support and fight for sex education programs, particularly those stressing the need for population control.
4. When the time comes for you to marry and have children, think about adopting a child rather than having one of your own.

Pertinent Facts

1. Population increases geometrically, so that the time needed for the population to double has gone from 1,500 years in 8,000 B.C. to 35 years in 1970.
2. The populations of developed countries are responsible for a major part of the resultant pollution through the use of large quantities of materials.
3. Population may be controlled by a number of contraceptive means, including both chemical and surgical.
4. Future contraceptive techniques may include long-term drugs and reversible surgical procedures which will be 100 percent effective and safe.
5. Government control of population could involve various forms of financial controls.

Possible Quiz

1. List three different ways in which contraception can be accomplished.
2. Historically, what were some of the controls on population growth that have now been overcome?
3. What are some sterilization operations? Do they affect sexuality? Why?
4. Why do many individuals and agencies feel that population control is essential to our survival?
5. What means could a government use to encourage voluntary limitation of family size?

READINGS

Berelson, Bernard, et al., *Family Planning and Population Programs.* Chicago: University of Chicago Press, 1966.

Davis, Kingsley, "Population," *Scientific American.* 209, September, 1963.

Guttmacher, Alan F., *The Complete Book of Birth Control.* New York: Ballantine Books, 1966.

Thompson, Warren S., and David J. Lewis, *Population Problems.* New York: McGraw-Hill Book Co., Inc., 1965.

FILMS

"Abortion and the Law." 54 minutes, sound, color, $15.00. Association Films, 600 Madison Avenue, New York, New York 10022.

"Multiply and Subdue the Earth." 15 minutes, sound, color, $18.00. Field Service, Indiana University, A-V Center, Bloomington, Indiana.

"People By the Billions." 28 minutes, sound, black and white, $8.00. McGraw-Hill Contemporary Film Rental Office, 330 West 42nd Street, New York, New York 10018.

Environment
and
Health

UNIT 5

LESSON 22

The Effects of
Alcohol on Human Tissue

Lesson time: 45 minutes

Aim

To provide the student with concrete evidence concerning the effects of alcohol consumption on the human body.

Materials

films

Planned Lesson

A study of alcohol's effects on the body can be used to begin a series of lessons dealing with various addictions which are prevalent in modern society. There is a great deal of confusion and misinformation about alcohol and its use. Some student suggestions of facts about alcohol can be elicited by the teacher. *Does alcohol stimulate the user? Is it a food? Is it an effective medicine for poor circulation?* Many other similar questions can be suggested by the teacher.

Students may have some experience with alcohol and can suggest some characteristic physiological reactions to it. They may suggest flushing, sensation of warmth, loss of efficiency, loss of voluntary muscle control leading to staggering and slurred speech, increased urination, euphoria, and impaired judgment. The teacher should then review the suggestions in an orderly pattern.

1. *Is Alcohol a Food?*   This commonly asked question provides a good point for reviewing some necessary biochemistry. The teacher may need to mention that drinking (ethyl) alcohol provides no nutritional material in the diet although it does provide calories. It needs no digestion and is quickly absorbed into the small intestine. Over ninety percent of the alcohol taken into the body will be disposed of by oxidation. An interesting point is that although the first step in alcohol breakdown (alcohol→acetaldehyde) occurs in the liver which is the only place where sufficient enzymes for the process are found, researchers generally do not believe that this is the way cirrhosis is caused; rather a faulty diet is more likely the cause.

Once again the students' reports, field trips, guest lectures, and films all provide valuable experiences. Reports on the number of drinkers in the United States (70 million of whom 5 million are considered alcoholics), Alcoholics Anonymous, and research on those who are likely to become alcoholics should be included. Other reports might provide biochemical information such as the fact that in a 150 pound person one-half to one fluid ounce of 100 proof alcohol is about completely oxidized in one hour. (One-half to one fluid ounce of 100 proof alcohol is about what is in one mixed drink or a 12 ounce can of beer.) *Why do articles and publicity campaigns recommend one drink per hour as a safe drinking rate?*

Can you speed up the oxidation of alcohol? Students may suggest increased exercise, going out in the cold, and a variety of home remedies, but actual clinical studies show that none of these work. There is some evidence that high levels of certain sugars in the body may increase the oxidation rate somewhat.

Can you slow down the absorption of alcohol? Here home remedies will include drinking olive or salad oil, eating ice cream, or ingesting other foods before drinking. Research has determined that absorption can be slowed and that pulpy food such as potatoes or a full meal are most effective.

2. *What Are the Specific Physiological Effects of Alcohol?* Now the class can consider the effects on the various systems and

organs of the body. Beginning with the superficial effects, they might analyze the flushing of the face and the general sensation of warmth. *Are the phenomena related? Is the room really warmer? Is the "drinker's nose" a real physiological phenomenon or just a cartoon representation?* The teacher might mention that in cases of drunken stupor the circulation would be impaired and the individual would be cold and pale.

Moving to the effects on the stomach, students may be familiar with the phenomenon of excessive drinking followed by vomiting. *Is this reaction a helpful one physiologically? What causes it?* If a guest lecturer is invited to class, he may also mention that heavy drinkers frequently suffer with chronic gastritis.

Virtually all students will have heard of cirrhosis of the liver as the scourge of heavy drinkers. An interested student might contact a local hospital or nursing school for permission to research this disease in their library. They will find that it is six times more common among heavy drinkers than in the general population and that it probably results from malnutrition. This in turn is caused by a reduced intake of food, with the calories supplied by alcohol. *Since alcohol does provide calories for energy production why would a diet of alcohol lead to malnutrition?*

Students may be aware that drinking increases urine output. The effect is on the pituitary gland whose function might briefly be reviewed here. It is not a valuable diuretic, however, because it does not cause a corresponding salt loss. (This may also provide a good point at which to review kidney function.)

For example, the process of urine formation can be studied in greater detail. Students should be able to trace the path of blood and the movement of liquids and nitrogenous wastes through the nephron, by using a diagram similar to Figure 22-1. They should pay special attention to the reabsorption of water, and to the distinctions between threshold or useful substances and nonthreshold substances. The teacher might provide students with a list of substances and ask them to categorize them. The list could include glucose, urea, amino acids, uric acid, sodium, and chloride ions. *At what point in the filtration process are ammonia and urea removed?*

Special student reports might be made on the antidiuretic

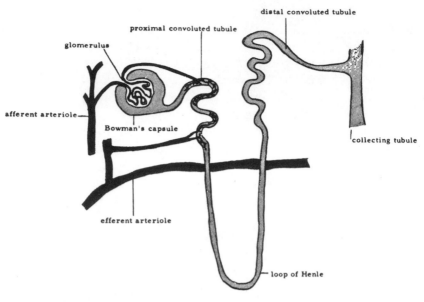

Figure 22-1. Nephron

hormone (ADH) and its relation to liquid intake and the amount
of urine voided; aldosterone; and other influencing factors, as well
as other topics of interest. *What characteristics of kidney function
make it possible for man to live in many different environments?*

Finally, the most important effects, those on the central
nervous system, can be considered. Here student suggestions will
have covered many of the phenomena. The teacher will have to
supply the physiological details. One point which should be
stressed is that despite popular belief, alcohol does not increase
efficiency, rather it lessens restraints. As little as 0.04% alcohol in
the blood can impair hearing and vision. Small amounts of alcohol,
even only one-half to one ounce can affect voluntary muscle
control because of interference with brain control. The range is
from slight impairment in intricate work to complete paralysis and
coma. As the percentage of alcohol in the blood reaches high
levels, involuntary muscles become involved. Death results from
respiratory failure preceded by very weak heart action. Probably
of most significance to the students is the impairment of brain

function in terms of voluntary muscle control, reaction time, and judgment. The highest brain functions, it should be stressed, are impaired at levels of lower alcohol concentration so that coordination would still be unaffected when judgment was already impaired. Euphoria is also a characteristic response. *In driving or hazardous work why would even a low alcohol level in the blood be dangerous? Why are chemical tests to determine driving under the influence of alcohol more meaningful than walking a straight line or other physical tests?* A student report might deal with the statistics of highway accidents and deaths related to drunken drivers.

3. *Diseases Related to Alcohol Consumption.* Included here might be cirrhosis, pancreatitis, alcoholic hallucinations, delirium tremens (DTs). Some symptoms of alcoholism can be mentioned. Malnutrition, coma, fatigue, chronic indigestion, jaundice, and convulsions would all be included. It is important for the teacher to point out that alcoholism is not restricted to the derelicts sometimes seen in city streets. Experts indicate that large numbers of alcoholics maintain jobs and may hold very important positions. The clue is whether they are addicted or not. That is, do they need a drink? Can they really not drink if they choose? As mentioned in the lesson on drugs, any chemical substance which becomes a necessity to body functions is an addictive substance. Students may be surprised to find many books and reports on addiction dealing with alcohol and drugs.

In mentioning the skid row alcoholics, the teacher may be asked about the dangers in drinking wood alcohol as is sometimes reported in the news. It might be valuable to trace the oxidation of methyl alcohol through its breakdown to formaldehyde and formic acid down to carbon dioxide and water. Generally, students know that formaldehyde is a powerful preservative and is very irritating to lungs and skin even with only superficial contact. Few may know that formic acid is a commonly used poison for native poison darts. *What might you predict about the effects of methyl alcohol oxidation products on cell physiology?*

Members of Alcoholics Anonymous make excellent speakers and can be contacted through the local chapter which is listed in the phone directory.

What Can You Do?

1. If you must drink, do not drink to excess. The recommended level of drinking is one drink per hour.
2. Low levels of alcohol consumption do impair those centers of the brain controlling judgment and reason. If you must drink, do so at home. Do not operate any vehicle while under the influence of alcohol.
3. Explain the effects of alcohol consumption to your parents and friends. This will help them to better understand what does (or does not) happen when one is under its influence.
4. A person who drinks a lot but does not eat well is prone to cirrhosis of the liver. If you must drink, make certain that you eat a well-balanced meal.

Pertinent Facts

1. Alcohol does not provide nutrition and is therefore not a food.
2. Alcohol in the blood affects higher brain functions, including reaction time and judgment, before physical effects can be identified.
3. Alcohol is an irritant which can cause stomach inflammation and vomiting.
4. It is extremely dangerous to drive or do hazardous work when drinking because of poor judgment and lack of coordination. Slowed reaction time and euphoria can lead to accidents and are dangerous because they occur before obvious physical effects.
5. Heavy drinking is associated with cirrhosis, pancreatitis, chronic gastritis, paralysis, nerve disorders, coma, and death.

Possible Quiz

1. Why does the intake of even a small amount of alcohol cause increased facial color and a sensation of warmth?

2. Is alcohol a food? Explain your answer.
3. Are there ways to slow alcohol absorption? What are they?
4. What system is most strongly affected by alcohol? What effects are involved?
5. Why is the expression "alcohol and gasoline don't mix" such an important one?

READINGS

Bier, William Christian, *Problems in Addiction: Alcohol and Drug Addiction.* New York: Fordham University Press, 1962.

"On Drunkenness," *Quarterly Journal of Studies of Alcohol.* New Brunswick, New Jersey: Rutgers Center for Alcohol Studies, 3:302-306, 1942.

Keeler, Mark (ed.), *International Bibliography of Studies on Alcohol.* New Brunswick, New Jersey: Rutgers Center for Alcohol Studies, 1966-1968.

McCarthy, Raymond G., *Alcohol Education for Classroom and Community.* New York: McGraw-Hill, 1964.

(The Rutgers Center has a wide range of publications in this field.)

FILMS

"Alcohol and the Human Body." 14 minutes, sound, black and white, $3.65. Encyclopedia Brittanica Educational Corporation, 425 North Michigan Avenue, Chicago, Ill. 60611.

"Alcoholism." 23 minutes, sound, black and white, $4.15. Encyclopedia Brittanica Educational Corporation, 425 North Michigan Avenue, Chicago, Ill. 60611.

LESSON 23

The Physiologic
Effects of Smoking

Lesson time: 45 minutes

Aim

To provide the student with concrete evidence concerning the harmful effects of smoking on the human body.

Materials

films

Planned Lesson

1. *Smoking and You.* As an introduction, the teacher might assign the reading of a book such as *The Consumers Union Report on Smoking and the Public Interest.* Although several years old, this report by a source which has a reputation for honest investigation is still excellent. The teacher might begin by discussing the increasing death rate due to lung cancer. Students are usually surprised to learn that it was once considered a rare disease.

Points to be stressed include the startling statistic that eighty to ninety percent of all inhaled cigarette smoke particles are retained by the lungs. In preparation for the lesson on emphysema it can be mentioned that lung irritation is directly responsible for emphysema. Student readings should provide specific information on carcinogens found in cigarettes. There are seven identified compounds in cigarettes which have caused cancer in laboratory animals. *Are laboratory animal experiments meaningful?* The many research projects on smoking suggest that smoke constituents are more damaging in combination than individually. Some researchers hypothesize that this may be related to physiological damage such as mucous membrane damage and interference with the ciliary transport mechanism. (If it is necessary, a review of respiratory system function might be appropriate here although a short explanation of the role of cilia will probably suffice.) Nine of the gases of cigarette smoke are lung irritants which also inhibit the action of cilia. *Specifically, how does smoking affect cilial action?* Discussion should emphasize that the number of ciliated cells decreases, the remaining cilia are shortened, and the mucous secreting cells are altered. Perhaps by reviewing the lesson on air pollution the teacher can remind the class that the cilia are important in keeping particles out of the lungs and that smoking and air pollution combine to increase lung irritation. *If cilia don't operate effectively, how is the individual in an air polluted area affected?*

2. *Why Is It that When One Stops Smoking Lung Function Improves?* Here the nature of alveolar phagocytes should be introduced. Students should understand that normally these phagocytes can ingest tobacco smoke components but they cannot keep up with increased levels caused by heavy smoking. When one stops smoking, these phagocytes can remove this material.

Again, the most effective class projects include preparing bulletin boards, school projects, visits by doctors, representatives of the Heart Association, Respiratory Disease Association, and perhaps field trips to hospital facilities.

3. *Some Smoking Statistics.* A display of compiled statistics would be an effective school project. Frequently, students direct vague references to statistics but are impressed by the staggering numbers actually involved. For example, there is a seventy percent higher death rate among male smokers than nonsmokers. Smoking five or more cigars per day increases the death rate over non-

smokers slightly, while pipe smokers have a death rate equal to nonsmokers. *How do numbers of cigarettes per day and numbers of years smoking affect death rate?*

4. *Relationship Between Smoking and Disease. What diseases would you think are related to smoking?* Advertising should have made students aware of the relationships between smoking and cardiovascular disease, coronary artery disease, chronic bronchitis, and emphysema. They may not be aware of the increased incidence of peptic ulcers among smokers or the fact that smoking during pregnancy causes lower birth weight in infants.

A review of the lesson will point out the indisputable evidence linking smoking and respiratory illness. Students might make a survey of the community to determine how many are smokers, how many are nonsmokers, and how many gave up smoking. *Have the public education campaigns been effective in your community?*

What Can You Do?

1. Inform your parents and friends of the statistics concerning smoking and decreased longevity, as well as the relationship between smoking and the incidence of various related diseases.
2. Smoking not only pollutes the atmosphere but your lungs as well. Give up smoking.

Pertinent Facts

1. There are a number of carcinogens in cigarette smoke and its particles.
2. Physiologic effects of smoking include damage to mucous membranes, cilia, and irritation to the entire respiratory complex.
3. A smoker living in an area of air pollution is doubly affected by the pollution because the smoking interferes with ciliary transport and thus more irritating particles are likely to enter the lungs.

4. The death rate for smokers in any age group is much higher than for the nonsmoker.
5. Smokers have higher rates of cardiovascular disease, coronary disease, and emphysema.

Possible Quiz

1. What conditions might be responsible for the increase in the once-rare lung cancer?
2. Identify some of the physiological "rewards" of smoking.
3. Explain the action of the tracheal cilia in the normal lung and compare with action in a smoker's lung.
4. What diseases have been linked with smoking?

READINGS

Consumers Union, "The Consumers Union Report on Smoking and the Public Interest," 1959.

U.S. Public Health Service, "The Surgeon-General's Advisory Committee on Smoking." No. 1103, January, 1964.

FILMS

"Smoking and You." 11 minutes, sound, color, $3.65. Indiana University, A-V Center, Bloomington, Indiana.

LESSON 24

Narcotics and
Their Effects

Lesson time: 90 minutes
Laboratory time: 90 minutes

Aim

To examine the various kinds of narcotics and to illustrate the physiological effects of drug abuse on man by observing changes in drugged water fleas in the laboratory.

Materials

films	microscopes
depression slides	culture of Daphnia
eyedroppers	antibiotics
antihistamine	amphetamine
aspirin	alcohol
barbiturate	coffee

Planned Lesson

1. *What Are Narcotics?* The lesson should cover both the beneficial and harmful aspects of drugs, although emphasis should be on their abuse. The class might begin with an attempt at listing those substances which are narcotics. Students will probably

suggest marijuana, LSD, heroin, amphetamines, and the many common medical preparations including sleeping pills and tran- quilizers.

The teacher will need to point out that not all drugs are narcotics. The name itself from "narcos," numbing, should help students come to an understanding of the classification. They might check a medical dictionary in order to understand that a narcotic is a substance which produces stupor or insensibility. Marijuana, for example, is not classified as a narcotic.

Student reports might focus on the number of drug users in the United States and other countries. They will learn that about five million Americans are considered to be alcoholics while seventy million use alcohol; that fifteen million use amphetamines, thirty million barbituates, and twelve million tranquilizers. There are over 50,000 hard-core heroin addicts in the country.

It would be wise to consider each drug separately. Students should be encouraged to read in advance about each drug. A great number of books, articles, and programs are devoted to drugs so that all should be able to obtain information.

2. *Marijuana.* Although not a narcotic, the widespread use of marijuana today and the many claims for and against it, suggest its inclusion here. Current references suggest that there are about six million marijuana users today. *What are the physiological effects of smoking marijuana?* Student research should have discovered that pulse rate and blood pressure increase, pupils dilate, lack of coordination, clumsiness and dry mouth are all effects. Decreased inhibitions, difficulty in concentration, diz- ziness, nausea, faintness and restlessness are also likely to occur.

Does it affect everyone in the same way? Students should seek out recent research information as part of their study. The teacher has a good opportunity here to stress the importance of critical analysis of facts rather than dependence on gossip or hearsay. They will discover that researchers indicate that person- ality plays a role in the effects marijuana has on individuals. Although euphoria is common and may last up to four or five hours, researchers note that people with psychological problems frequently are adversely affected. *Do you think the physical and psychological stresses of adolescence might cause specific effects?* Here the teacher might introduce the idea that one school of thought is that simply by being an adolescent one already has a number of stress factors working on him which can be intensified by marijuana use.

A deeper study will indicate that generally when one smokes marijuana he does not engage in physical activity, perhaps because of the dizziness and clumsiness it causes. The more complex functions of the brain are most seriously affected. Recent findings suggest that products of marijuana metabolism may be found in the body a year after the last time it was smoked. The teacher may or may not want to explore the various views on marijuana smoking and its relationship to use of other drugs. If this is covered, ample material is available in books and periodicals for student research. The psychological factors which act to influence marijuana should be considered and compared with factors which might influence the use of other drugs.

3. *LSD.* Lysergic acid diethylamide can be considered next. It is valuable to discuss the "set" and "setting" referred to by researchers. The "set" or frame of mind and "setting" or environment in which LSD is taken have been identified in clinical studies. LSD is considered to be the most powerful psychedelic drug known. Students can gather information from books and periodicals and from local drug programs. Perhaps a visiting lecturer can be invited to class from one of these groups. LSD "trips" vary depending on set, setting, and dosage. Reactions range from increased sensitivity to stimuli to emergence of subconscious, to what is described as mystical and religious experiences. The drug is so potent that one writer suggests that thirty-five pounds of it could "turn on" the entire country. After taking LSD, response begins within fifteen minutes to one hour. A trip lasts eight to ten hours, generally reaching full intensity in about one and one-half hours. After about four hours the effects begin to decrease in intensity.

How does LSD work? Students will discover that the specific action of LSD is on the diencephalon or midbrain. *How does this relate to the effects of LSD use?* The teacher should point out that the midbrain controls emotional response, consciousness, many physiological functions (including pupil contraction and temperature). It should also be pointed out that the individual quickly develops a tolerance for the drug.

What about bad trips? The earlier information on set should be brought in here as should the release of the subconscious and diencephalon control of emotions. The possibility of feelings of serious danger, bleeding to death, severe wounds, or other terrifying experiences are all common. Students must realize that such reactions can't be predicted. These and other sensations have been known to cause individuals to take their own lives while tripping. It will also be important to mention the recurrence of trips without additional use of LSD. *What possible reasons can you give for this?* It must also be mentioned that LSD causes chromosome breakage. The teacher may wish to review DNA briefly here.

Students should be reminded that a chromosome is actually a single molecule of deoxyribonucleic acid (DNA). Building on your students' knowledge of the Watson-Crick model of DNA, as illustrated in Figure 24-1, you can begin to explain the theory as it relates to coding. In this manner, the concept that a series of bases arranged in a sequential pattern are the segments of chromosomes which are called genes, can be developed. These genes control all metabolic functioning of the cell. It should be made clear that the arrangement of bases along the molecule can have many variations. Students should be encouraged to consider possible consequences of these variations. Investigators believe that reading down the DNA molecule three bases at a time provides the code. These three base groups are known as triplets or codons. Thus, it can now be seen that genes are simply a series of codons. *What might happen if a drug such as LSD caused a break in the DNA molecule?*

4. *Heroin.* The various derivatives of opium might be used to introduce the study of heroin. These include the milder drug paregoric which is used for stomach upsets as well as being the commonly prescribed teething medication for babies. Codeine, another opiate, may be familiar as a component of common cough medicines. *Why are codeine containing drugs specially controlled in some states?* The common pain killer, Demerol, can also be

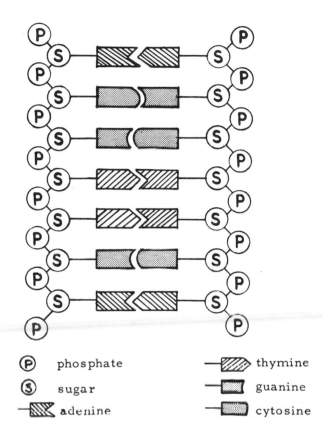

Figure 24-1. DNA Structure Model

mentioned here as a man-made drug similar to the opiates. Finally, heroin and morphine can be studied as the most powerful opium derivatives. *Why are doctors careful about prescribing morphine even though it is a very effective painkiller?*

Methods of use. A great many students have some knowledge of the slang of drug users. They know that heroin is "scag," junk, horse, H, or other terms and they may have heard about snorting, skin-popping and mainlining. It is important that these be reviewed because all too often students think that only injecting into a vein or mainlining is dangerous.

Actually "snorting" or inhaling heroin has been known to cause death. Physiologically it is no less addicting than any other method. Heroin is readily absorbed into the blood through the nasal membranes.

"Skin-popping" or injecting heroin under the skin is the usual next stage in heroin use, but because the body builds tolerance to heroin quickly, even this method is ultimately too slow and so the user moves on to "mainlining." *What happens when heroin enters the body?* Students would probably gain from having a doctor who is involved in heroin addict treatment programs come to the school to discuss addiction and answer questions. It is important that someone actually involved in drug work be asked since students will not relate to an individual who speaks unrealistically from a sideline position. They will usually be quite enthusiastic with someone who has firsthand experience and be more likely to accept what is said. The teacher must also realize that it is likely that some of the students may be closely associated with drug users or may be users themselves. It is vital that drug material be presented logically, not irrationally. The need is to have students really listen and be willing to accept the presented facts.

Physiological reactions to heroin should be considered. As has been suggested, mainlining is the fastest way to get a heroin response. It is estimated that reaction occurs within one minute of injection. Soon after, drowsiness occurs. *What does "on the nod" suggest?* This is a characteristic by which the seemingly napping addict can be identified. When the drowsiness begins to wear off, it's time to plan for getting the next of what may be three or four fixes a day. *What are the effects of heroin use?* Students might be surprised to discover that no organic damage has been identified as typical of heroin addiction. As is true of all addictions including alcohol, the body does become chemically dependent on heroin. There *are* many harmful effects of heroin addiction. From communal use of needles, addicts frequently develop hepatitis, collapsed veins, abscesses and even fatal tetanus. Because addicts are usually indifferent to food, they suffer from malnutrition and are susceptible to pneumonia. Since it is an opiate and painkiller, the heroin makes a user less sensitive to pain and so he may easily injure himself. Overdoses of heroin are fatal. In New York City more deaths of young people occur from heroin than all contagious diseases combined. This tragic statistic reflects a nationwide pattern.

An important effect of heroin addiction is the altered behavior it necessitates. Although it has been shown that heroin does not cause criminal behavior, the addict exhibits criminal behavior generally because it is necessary to continuously get money (perhaps as much as $150 per day) to support the addiction.

Perhaps student groups could research and prepare displays dealing with drug programs such as Synanon, Phoenix House, Odyssey House and many others. It is important to point out the addicts who wish to be helped can be helped and that today there are many ex-addicts leading normal lives.

5. *Other Drugs.* Here the teacher might review STP (2,5 dimethyl-4-methyl amphetamine) said to be stronger than LSD. This hallucinogen produces three- to four-day trips which may be horrifying. It is a particularly dangerous drug because it cannot be taken with other drugs. Drug users are known to use tranquilizers and sedatives to calm down an LSD high. When this is tried with STP its physiological effects on the central nervous system are intensified. This frequently results in death, impaired breathing, irregular heart beat, or nerve damage.

DMT, called the "lunch hour special," is a hallucinogen which produces results within seconds. The high usually lasts from fifteen to thirty minutes.

A large variety of other substances have been used to get high. Glue sniffing, students should note, causes serious damage to kidney and liver cells and may also cause dizziness, unconsciousness, and fatal coma. *What special danger is involved in not being able to control dosage?* Amylnitrite, a heart and asthma drug, increases circulation. *Why is it used along with hallucinogens?* The discussion might conclude with the study of aerosol quick freeze substances sometimes sold for chilling cocktail glasses or similar uses. Deaths have resulted from sniffing this material, actually Freon 12. Autopsy showed death by asphyxiation due to a frozen larynx.

Speed. (Methedrine, crystal or methamphetamine hydro-chloride.) *Why is it called "speed"?* This drug's very quick action affects the central nervous system. Nicknames such as lid-proppers, eyeopeners, and copilots all suggest its use by truck drivers, for example, to keep awake. Many other nicknames relate to the chemical name or appearance of amphetamines. "Bennies" are benzedrine, "dexies," dexedrine. *Is speed addicting?* Student research will indicate that the drugs are not physically addicting but may be said to cause psychological addiction. Accentuating psychological problems, speed can cause insanity. Chronic use causes brain damage, memory loss, violence. Because "coming down" is bad, users tend to try to stay up. "Speed kills," the popular slogan, suggests the high number of deaths among its users.

Finally the terms "ups and downs" should be considered with a discussion of depressants and stimulants. If available, a local pharmacologist might present a lecture on drugs.

Although a great many films on drug abuse are available they *must* be carefully previewed in advance. Some are so poorly done that they may seriously interfere with the rapport the teacher has developed with the students. Such rapport is crucial if students are to accept what the teacher presents to them and it may also encourage students to seek the teacher's help with their own drug problems.

Laboratory Activity

Students can determine the effects of various classes of drugs on the heart and circulatory system by using an easily observable laboratory animal such as Daphnia (water flea). These can be obtained from commercial suppliers or from tropical fish stores, and should be kept in an isolated aquarium. Figure 24-2 can be used to identify the heart of this organism.

The teacher should obtain one sample of a number of different classes of substances, such as a barbiturate, ampheta-mine, antihistamine, mild narcotic such as found in cough syrup, antibiotic, aspirin, alcohol, and coffee. Drugs which require pre-scriptions can be obtained from the school or family physician. By preparing water solutions of these in varying strengths, students

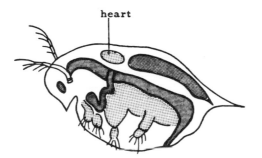

Figure 24-2. Daphnia

can investigate the effects of different concentrations of these on the heart.

The Daphnia should be transferred from the culture bottle to a depression slide by means of an eyedropper. There should be only enough water on the slide to keep the Daphnia alive. The Daphnia should then be observed under low power, with special attention being given to the rapidly beating heart.

Be sure to time the heartbeat for one minute *before* you add your test solution. *Why?* Place a drop of one of the solutions on the Daphnia. *What is the effect on the heart?* By repeating this procedure with the remaining solutions, the effects of stimulants, depressants, and other materials on the heart can be seen. Each group of students may be assigned a single drug, or if a sufficient number of Daphnia are available, each group may test a number of different solutions. *Why is it necessary to use a fresh specimen for each test? Why are Daphnia well suited to this activity?*

What Can You Do?

1. Unless prescribed by a doctor for medical reasons do not take drugs of any kind.
2. Most drugs are not only addicting, but can cause serious physiological harm and may even lead to death.
3. If you know someone who is a drug user, try to get him to seek professional help to "kick the habit."

4. Report to your parents or proper school authorities any person whom you know or suspect of selling drugs to your friends and other students.

Pertinent Facts

1. There are millions of drug abusers in the United States.
2. Much more research is needed to establish whether marijuana may be injurious. It is not considered to be narcotic.
3. LSD, DMT, and STP all are hallucinogens which can cause bad trips and may lead to death, chromosome damage, and recurring trips.
4. Heroin addiction is a very serious condition which usually results in the necessity of committing criminal acts. It may also involve hepatitis, malnutrition, pneumonia, and serious injury.
5. Amphetamines cause many deaths as well as many cases of brain damage and memory loss.

Possible Quiz

1. Identify three drugs widely used today and give some examples of their effects on the human body.
2. What complications commonly occur from the injection of a drug?
3. Why is it particularly dangerous to use central nervous system depressants along with STP?
4. What are some effects of LSD? Why do some people have bad trips? What specifically are the physiological effects of LSD on the body?
5. Using the physiological effects it causes as the basis of your answer, explain why the slogan says, "Speed Kills."

READINGS

Geller, Allen and Maxwell Boac, *The Drug Beat.* New York: Cowles, 1969.

Leech, Kenneth and Brenda Jordan, *Drugs for Young People: Their Use and Misuse.* Oxford, England: Pergammon Press, 1967.

You, Your Child, and Drugs. Washington, D.C.: Child Study Association of America, 1971.

It would be impossible to provide a definitive list of sources. Teachers should check lists of new books, publications, and book reviews for new references.

Contact the National Clearinghouse for Drug Abuse Information or local programs. Be sure to preview in advance as suggested earlier.

Educational materials can be obtained from: Child Study Association of America, Lillian Opatoshu, Program Director, 9 East 89th Street, New York, New York 10028.

FILMS

"Drug Addiction." 22 minutes, sound, black and white, $4.15. Encyclopedia Britannica Films, Inc., 1150 Wilmette Avenue, Wilmette, Illinois 60091.

"Hooked." 28-31 minutes, sound, black and white, free loan. Narcotic Addiction Control Commission, Executive Park South, Albany, New York 12203.

"The Losers." 28-31 minutes, sound, color, free loan. Narcotic Control Commission.

"Narcotics: Why Not?" 15 minutes, sound, color, free loan. Narcotic Addiction Control Commission.

"The Seekers," 30 minutes, sound, color, free loan. Narcotic Addiction Control Commission.

LESSON 25

Infectious Diseases

Lesson time: 90 minutes
Laboratory time: 45 minutes

Aim

To examine laboratory cultures of microorganisms and relate disease-causing pathogens to the major communicable diseases of man with an emphasis on their treatment and prevention.

Materials

> nonpathogenic bacteria
> slides of pathogens
> microscopes

Planned Lesson

1. *What Causes Disease?*   Discussion can begin with the germ theory of disease and a brief introduction to microorganisms. The types of organisms, according to shape, should be mentioned, including bacilli or rods, spirella or spirals, and cocci or spherical organisms. Staphylococci, the *grape cluster-like* organism, and streptococci, the *chain-like* organism, might be specifically mentioned since they are well known. If the teacher would like to provide some microbiological technique practice, students can collect nonpathogenic bacteria from any decaying matter. A good

classroom source would be a vase of flowers in which the water has not recently been changed. Sauerkraut juice and yoghurt are other sources. Simple wet mounts may be used for observation. (For this and more advanced techniques see Lesson 1.) For students interested in culturing bacteria, the teacher can suggest basic references such as those in the bibliography. It is extremely important that such work be carefully supervised. Certainly no pathogens should be cultured, but some may be inadvertently grown if careless techniques allow for contamination. When students are not practiced at sterile technique such contamination is not unusual. Accuracy of technique *must* be carefully supervised.

In the laboratory the students might use microscopes to observe prepared slides of pathogens in each group. They will be able to observe the general shape of each as well as to study the specific organism itself. Perhaps the teacher can integrate lecture and laboratory so that a brief introduction to each disease or group of diseases can be followed by laboratory observation and questions.

2. *Respiratory Disease.* Work might begin with the discussion of chronic versus acute. Here the lesson on emphysema can be tied in. Student suggestions might include chronic emphysema, bronchitis, and cancers, while acute illnesses would be flu, pneumonia, measles, mumps, mononucleosis, and rubella.

The interrelations of disease to environment and culture should be stressed. *What are some factors believed to be involved in development of emphysema, bronchitis, and lung cancer?* This will help to connect the lessons on air pollution, smoking, and emphysema. *How do cultural pressure and public information campaigns affect attitudes toward chronic respiratory diseases and medical treatment?* Here the whole gamut of ecological problems can be interrelated.

3. *Infectious Diseases.* Measles, mumps, and rubella can be the center of a discussion on inoculation campaigns and the great changes in societies as effective vaccines are developed to prevent disease. It should be stressed that diseases which we think of as "harmless" because they are common can be fatal. Perhaps students can collect pamphlets on each of the diseases and prepare a display for a school bulletin board. *Why is rubella so dangerous to*

pregnant women? A very interesting lecture could be arranged with the local public health authorities or those of a nearby city. The problems of public education, for example, can be complex. *How can a campaign educate children to the need for vaccinations without appearing to suggest that the parents are ignorant?* New York City's "Rubella Umbrella" commercials, for example, provide children with the basic information on the need for rubella vaccination and where to get it in such a way that the child will then tell the parents without offending them in any way. The ramifications of such advertising can be fully explored. *Why are they an important part of public health programs?*

Influenza and the 1916 epidemic provides another aspect of study. *Why was the 1916 episode called a pandemic?* If students are encouraged to ask their parents about it, they are likely to find that members of their own family were lost. Here the teacher should stress scientific advances which provide vaccines, antibiotics and other weapons to fight disease, which were not always available. *Why are there strict international controls on such things as smallpox vaccination?* This also leads to the problem of increasing population.

Other infectious diseases can illustrate further aspects of environmental effects on health. *Why are there outbreaks of meningitis in large military camps?* Here the obvious connection between a large population in a limited space and the necessary close contact can suggest the ease with which highly contagious diseases spread. Tuberculosis and diphtheria would be included here. The main diseases carried by parasites again show the interrelations of environment and health. The use of human waste as fertilizer in some countries and the resultant spread of parasite eggs can be traced. Here ascaris, hookworm, and filarial worms can be used as examples. Charts showing their life cycles might be made. *How is malaria spread? How can it be controlled?*

4. *Communicable Diseases.* There is a great need for special emphasis on the communicable diseases directly related to the so-called "youth culture." The transmission of infectious hepatitis through use of contaminated hypodermic needles has caused many deaths among drug users. The epidemic of venereal diseases should be thoroughly studied. Statistics can be obtained from the U.S.

Public Health Service, Communicable Disease Center, Atlanta, Georgia. Charts and pamphlets are available from the U.S. Government Printing Office, Washington, D.C. 20025. It would be wise to seek the most recent information on this since the number of cases is constantly changing. Many areas of the United States have seen increases in venereal disease of 200 percent or more within the last few years.

It would be wise to review human anatomy and physiology briefly as a basis for the discussion. Because there is such an epidemic, class time should be given to a specific study of both syphilis and gonorrhea. The teacher may wish to make research of the subject a class project, but should be certain that specifics are thoroughly covered. Students need to know that the spirillum, Treponema pallidum, cannot survive outside the body unless maintained in a proper environment. Therefore objects which might be contaminated with syphilitic secretum will not be dangerous once the secretions dry (about one hour). The course of syphilis should be traced including incubation time from exposure (almost always through sexual intercourse although kissing someone with a chancre of the mouth might spread it) to development of chancre—2-6 weeks; primary stage—from appearance of chancre (ulcer) to systemic involvement—8-12 weeks; secondary stage—lesions may occur over period of 5 years; latent stage—no obvious signs for a few months or a whole lifetime but usually 6-7 years; tertiary stage—lesions of deeper structures of the body, particularly the cardiovascular and central nervous systems.

A particularly tragic aspect of the disease is the possibility of syphilis being passed on to the fetus during pregnancy. Complicating this is the fact that the chancre is usually on the cervix of a female so that she is not aware of its presence. (In most males, the chancre appears in the area of the genitalia, but in any case is external and visible during the primary stage.) A child of a syphilitic mother may not suffer from congenital syphilis at all, may have it at birth or develop it soon after, or may be born dead. Congenital syphilis involves skin lesions, nasal discharge, poorly developed permanent teeth, and the appearance of an old man.

It would be extremely valuable for the teacher to seek out a local resource person to give a lecture on the subject after class study to insure that the students will understand the basics.

Gonorrhea is a second epidemic problem today. It is the most prevalent infectious disease in the United States. Many misconceptions about gonorrhea circulate so that students believe it is not a very serious problem. The Public Health Service estimates that there are about four million cases a year. Students should understand that gonorrheal salpingitis is an oviduct infection. It causes scarring and blockage. In a similar infection in the male, scarring sequence occurs in the vasa deferentia. *Why is gonorrhea a major cause of sterility?* Gonorrhea can be transmitted to the victim's eyes quite easily. Virtually all states require routine treatment of newborn infants' eyes to prevent possible gonorrheal infection.

In summarizing the lesson, the teacher can stress the environmental factors of disease communication and control with specific emphasis on the epidemic of venereal diseases.

What Can You Do?

1. Inform your parents and friends about the environmental factors of disease communication and control, with specific emphasis on the epidemic of venereal disease.
2. Make certain that you, your parents, and friends have all your required inoculations and vaccinations.

Pertinent Facts

1. Diseases are caused by microorganisms which live and grow in a suitable environment.
2. Public education campaigns are important in disease control because they encourage people to be vaccinated and to seek prompt medical help for illness.
3. Infectious diseases can be controlled by inoculation or vaccination, medication, and by interrupting the life cycle of causative agents. This includes control of carriers such as insects and rodents.
4. Population increase aids in the spread of disease because of close contact.

5. An epidemic of venereal disease is now sweeping the United States, causing pain, illness, and death.

Possible Quiz

1. Identify and describe the major types of bacteria.
2. Give examples of five carriers of disease.
3. Discuss some of the ways in which the spread of disease can be controlled.
4. Describe the means of infection, course of disease, and damage caused by the venereal diseases syphilis and gonorrhea.
5. Explain why infection with either of these may not be treated or reported.

READINGS

Baker, Bill and Helen Kotsonis, *Modern Lesson Plans for the Biology Teacher.* West Nyack, N.Y.: Parker Publishing Co., Inc., 1970.

Brock, Thomas D., *Biology of Microorganisms.* Englewood Cliffs, N.J.: Prentice-Hall, Inc., 1970.

Eklund, Curtis and Charles E. Lankford, *Laboratory Manual for General Microbiology,* Englewood Cliffs, N.J.: Prentice-Hall, Inc., 1967.

Jawetz, Ernest, Joseph L. Melnick, and Edward A. Adelberg, *Review of Medical Microbiology,* 9th edition, Los Altos, California: Lange Medical Publication, 1970.

Smith, Alice Lorraine, *Microbiology and Pathology,* 9th edition, Saint Louis: C.V. Mosby Company, 1968.

FILMS

"Bacteria." 15 minutes, sound, color, $5.65. Indiana University, A-V Center, Bloomington, Indiana.

"Infectious Disease and Man-Made Defenses." 11 minutes, sound, color, $3.65. Coronet Films, Coronet Building, Chicago, Illinois 60601.

"Infectious Disease and Natural Body Defenses." 11 minutes, sound, color $3.65. Coronet Films.

LESSON 26

Emphysema

Lesson time: 45 minutes

Aim

To acquaint the student with basic information on emphysema, and to explore its relationship to air pollution and smoking.

Materials

films

Planned Lesson

1. *What Parts of the Body Does Emphysema Affect?*   The teacher might begin by reviewing the physiology of the human respiratory system. Students should be familiar with the anatomy of the human respiratory system, including the ciliated cells of the trachea, goblet cells, mucous membrane, bronchioles, and alveoli.

General statistics concerning the characteristic victim—male, white, between fifty and seventy years of age, and usually a *heavy smoker*—should be introduced. An interesting unexplained statistic should be mentioned and perhaps some theories can be developed by students. This is that men are ten times more likely to develop emphysema than women.

A very effective bulletin board display can be prepared

showing a sketch, such as Figure 26-1, of the respiratory system with inserts of enlarged sketches of those structures involved in emphysema. Pamphlets can be obtained from the National Tuberculosis Association, insurance companies, and other related organizations.

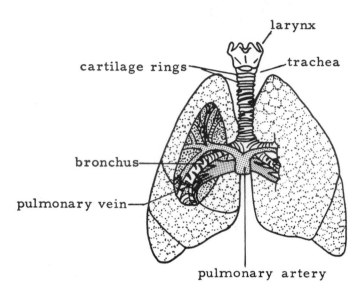

Figure 26-1. Respiratory System

Why do emphysema victims usually discover this condition after it is advanced? The creeping nature of the advance of this disease should be noted. Some symptoms include repeated heavy winter colds, a heavy cough, chronic bronchitis, and shortness of breath. *Considering the symptoms, why might someone not suspect he was suffering from emphysema?*

2. *Physiology of Emphysema.* The teacher should point out that emphysema is a late result of chronic infection or irritation of the bronchial tubes. The irritation blocks airways, causing air to be trapped. The walls of the alveoli may then tear. *What effect do damaged alveoli and blocked airways have on external respiration?* Here the teacher can review the physiology of gas exchange, emphasizing the effect of decreased contact of air on the blood

capillaries. The discussion should go on to explain that continued stretching, damage, and infection will result in stretching of the entire lung. As a result, oxygen-carbon dioxide exchange is impaired.

3. *Can Emphysema Be Treated?* Students should be encouraged to use their knowledge of the physiological aspects of emphysema to suggest possible treatment. It should be obvious that control of infection would be important. The teacher should emphasize that the damage already done cannot be reversed.

The teacher might mention that, although the cause has not yet been identified, it is quite clear that heavy smokers are much more susceptible to emphysema than nonsmokers. Students might refer to the Report of the Surgeon General's Advisory Committee of Smoking for specific details.

What Can You Do?

1. Stop smoking—heavy smokers are much more susceptible to emphysema than nonsmokers.
2. If you have shortness of breath, heavy winter colds and chronic bronchitis, go for a checkup. You may be suffering from emphysema.

Pertinent Facts

1. Men are much more likely to develop emphysema than women. Smokers have a higher rate of incidence of emphysema than nonsmokers.
2. Emphysema is the result of chronic irritation and causes damage to bronchioles and alveoli.
3. Because the early symptoms include bronchitis and shortness of breath, emphysema sufferers may not realize that they have it.
4. Emphysema causes a reduction in exchange of oxygen and carbon dioxide during external respiration.
5. Although the damage cannot be undone, further damage can be prevented by eliminating the infection or irritation.

Possible Quiz

1. Describe a likely emphysema victim.
2. What causes emphysema and what damage does it produce?
3. What are some of the symptoms of emphysema?
4. How does emphysema affect the physiology of the human body?
5. What might an individual do to reduce the likelihood of developing emphysema?

READINGS

Anthony, C.A., *Textbook of Anatomy and Physiology.* St. Louis: C.V. Mosby, Co., 1969.

National Tuberculosis Association, "Emphysema: The Facts," 1965.

Pace, O., and B.W. McCashland, *College Physiology.* New York: Thomas Y. Crowell Co., 1966.

LESSON 27

Cancer

Lesson Time: 45 minutes

Aim

To familiarize the student with the physiological aspects of cancer, its causes, treatment, and common misconceptions about the disease.

Materials

films

Planned Lesson

1. *What Is Cancer?* The teacher might begin with a class discussion about the nature of cancer. Students will probably identify types of cancer including lung, skin, stomach, ovarian, rectal, leukemia, and bone cancer. This can be used to show that actually cancer is many different diseases, not really one at all. A review of cell structure and physiology would be helpful at this point. It should be stressed that normal growth provides for constant repair and replacement of cells as well as production of new organisms and that this growth rate is believed to be controlled by the genetic code. Abnormal growth of cells, which may serve as a definition of cancer, seems to be without purpose

207

in the physiology of the cell. The teacher might now distinguish between the terms "benign" and "malignant," noting that abnormal growth may produce a large number of cells, or tumor, which appear to be the same as the other cells of the tissue from which they grew. They develop the same pattern of cells within the tissue but there is an unusually large number of them. Benign tumors generally do not endanger life. The teacher might want to add here that although not dangerous itself, it might possibly cause pressure or blockage of some organ or organ part which could create a dangerous situation. An interested student might give an oral report on benign tumors including the fact that they are usually clearly separated from surrounding tissue by a layer of cells. This makes removal easier and also suggests the fact that such tumors do not metastasize (spread).

Malignant tumors might be the subject of another report. These are very different from surrounding cells, not well organized in the tissue, seem to be immature cells, and grow and spread rapidly. Some emphasis on spread of cancer from its original site must be included. Here it is important to stress the importance of early diagnosis so that students will understand the tragedy of delay in getting medical treatment.

The nature of cancer spread can be traced from the original wild divisions (for which there are as yet no definitive explanations), to the extension of rays of cells into surrounding tissue, and finally to the idea of metastasis, that is, the movement of cancer cells in the lymph or blood so that new areas of the body are invaded and cancerous divisions begin elsewhere. This pathway from primary **to** secondary cancers can be used as an excellent illustration of the need for early medical treatment.

Although no "cure" for all cancers has been found, many of the various types of cancer are considered curable or at least can be arrested. Only recently, specialists announced that leukemia can be considered to be a curable cancer. Students should be encouraged to develop reports on cancer research. They will be surprised at the number of cancers which are curable and the high rate of success in many cases, if treated early. It might be necessary to remind students that "curable" does not mean all victims survive any more than do all pneumonia victims survive. *What does curable mean?*

2. *Has the Cancer Death Rate Increased?*   Many students have heard comments about how many more people die of cancer today than in earlier times. They should investigate this belief. *How does record keeping affect death rate?* Students should consider the completeness of record keeping for cause of death in the United States and throughout the world. Perhaps a student could contact the local coroner, hospital, or Bureau of Vital Statistics for information. *Are deaths from cancer recorded as such or is the specific cause of death listed?* They may be surprised to discover that many death certificates list the specific lung, heart, or brain malfunction which caused clinical death and not the cancer which caused that malfunction. Another obvious factor is age. Since greater numbers of people are saved from death due to other illnesses, they live to develop cancer. Those people who died in the 1916 flu pandemic certainly did not live to develop cancer and so the rate may have been much lower for all those people dying at that time. Low cancer rates in many South American and Asian countries have been attributed to the very short life spans in these countries. Thus, better records and longer life, together with better diagnoses, all contribute to a larger number of identifiable cases of cancer.

3. *Causes of Cancer.*   Lesson 23 considered some of the interrelations of smoking and cancer. In a study of environment, it is important to identify those things which have been found to cause cancer. The teacher should point out that the "how" is what researchers feel will be the clue to prevention. This study might begin with an explanation that there is little evidence to suggest any patterns of heredity in cancer development although a few rare cancers are known to be hereditary.

Because of the well publicized Pap smear test, students may be familiar with the notion of precancerous conditions. Warnings about changes in moles are also involved in this aspect of cancer. They should be aware of the existence of certain conditions which are not cancerous themselves, but are known to be conditions which frequently lead to cancer. Here again, public fears should be stressed. The woman who is advised that the Pap test indicates a precancerous infection must realize that time is crucial.

Specifically linked to environmental study is the development of cancer due to irritation of tissue. Here we include lip cancer seen in men who continually have a pipe in the corner of the mouth, cigarette smokers who irritate the delicate lung with heat and chemicals, chronic infections of some organs, parasitic irritations, and other types of chronic, long-term irritation.

Viruses and their possible connection with cancer can be linked to various research reports students may have read in news media. The teacher might mention that many research institutions require elaborate precautions to prevent transmission of such viruses, if they exist.

Interested students can research misconceptions about cancer, beginning with family and friends. The various beliefs should be presented to the group and discussed. Frequently library research will be needed to ascertain whether the belief is fact or fallacy.

4. *How Is Cancer Treated?*   The various forms of treatment should be presented and discussed. These include surgical removal, radiation therapy, and chemotherapy. A specialist in the field could provide a valuable class experience. Perhaps a field trip to a laboratory or hospital could be arranged. Large cities frequently have a variety of specialized cancer facilities. The local chapter of the American Cancer Society can provide information on facilities, pamphlets, and available films.

Some time should be spent on discussion of quack treatments. Students should be helped to see that this tragic and frequently prolonged disease provides lucrative ground for fraud as well as for false hopes for untried or useless medication. The story of Krebiozen, for example, can be researched by the class. They should seek news information of the early 1960's. Many other "cancer cure" stories are available in the literature.

Interested students can go on to study the specific types of cancer, new research studies, or other related information.

What Can You Do?

1. If you have a mole which has increased in size or changed in color, go to your physician for a check-up. It may be nothing serious, but the sooner you go the better off you will be.

2. Go to your doctor at least once a year for a thorough

physical examination. Half the battle with cancer lies in its early detection.
3. Advise your parents and friends to have yearly physicals.

Pertinent Facts

1. Cancer is the abnormal growth of cells producing a tumor which may be benign or malignant.
2. Benign tumors grow slowly and are usually harmless although their presence may interfere with surrounding organs or cause pressure, such as on the brain.
3. Early detection and treatment of cancer is vital because it eventually invades surrounding tissue and may metastasize or be carried to other areas of the body.
4. Cancer may be caused by irritation, viruses, radiation, smoking, air pollution, or certain chemicals.
5. Cancer is treated by surgical removal, radiation therapy, and drugs

Possible Quiz

1. Explain how benign and malignant tumors differ.
2. Why is early detection of cancer important to successful treatment?
3. Identify some of the conditions which seem to cause cancer.
4. Describe the ways in which cancer is treated.
5. Discuss the psychological factors involved in avoidance of diagnosis and treatment when cancer is suspected and show how this develops into a cyclic phenomenon.

READINGS

Cameron, Charles S., *The Truth About Cancer*. New York: Macmillan, 1967.
Case, James F. and Vernon E. Stiers, *Biology Observation and Concept*. New York: Macmillan, 1971.

FILMS

"Cancer." 13 minutes, sound, black and white. $2.15. Encyclopedia Britannica Educational Corporation, 425 North Michigan Avenue, Chicago, Illinois 60611.

"Virus: Cancer." 29 minutes, sound, black and white, $5.40. Indiana University, A-V Center, Bloomington, Indiana.

Index

213

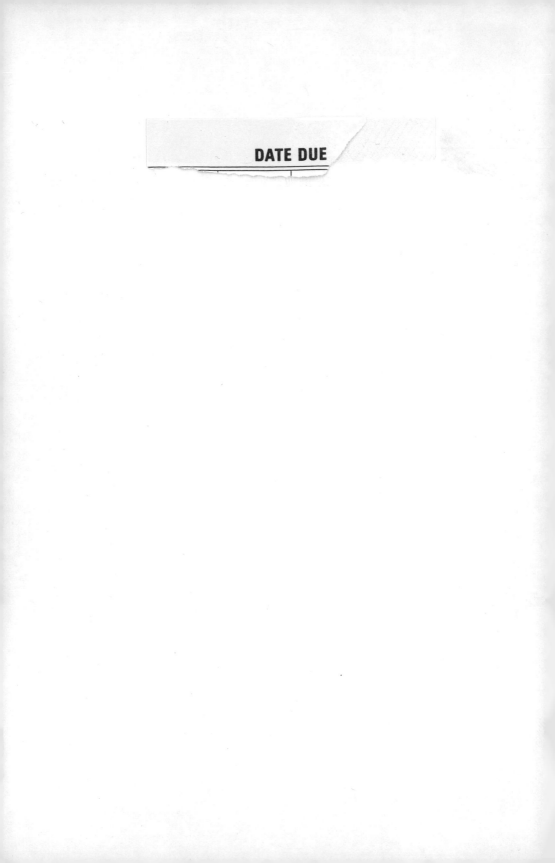

DATE DUE